Contents

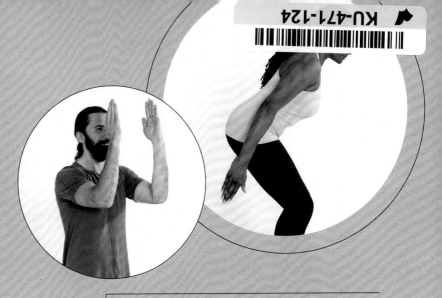

Introduction

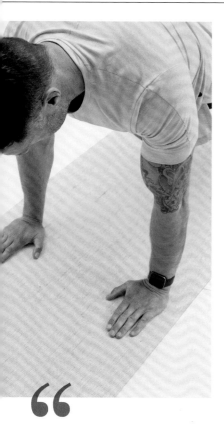

In this book, we hope to show you that enjoying good health and staying fit does not require hours in the gym. You can achieve this by moving more and, importantly, moving well, throughout your day.

The Pilates Express® programme has around 40 mini workouts, each designed for a specific part of your day: morning, midday and evening. The exercises, many brand new to Pilates, will make a huge difference to how you look and how you feel. But, perhaps most important of all, they will help you to stay healthy. We aim to restore balance in your body, making it resilient, flexible and strong enough, physically, mentally and emotionally, to tackle whatever life has in store.

Probably the single biggest obstacle to exercising regularly is lack of time. Setting aside an hour for a class may seem impossible, but ten minutes? That is surely doable. We show you simple ways to include more physical activity in your day, without having to schedule 'exercise sessions'. Perfect for those of you who are intention rich, time poor! Our goal is to use the mini workouts to reset and rebalance your body. And, because balance in your body requires balance in your life, we'll also look at small lifestyle changes that deliver big results.

MAXIMUM RESULTS IN MINIMUM TIME

The Pilates Express® programme will improve your strength and flexibility, toning every inch, streamlining your body. The exercises work on your posture, core stability and improve the efficiency of your breathing. These are things that Pilates is already famous for, but this time we are going further, deeper. We're also going to look at simple ways to ensure your body can cope with stress better, explore ways to reduce chronic inflammation (a major cause of many diseases) and help your immune system function optimally.

If lack of time is not your obstacle to exercising, maybe lack of motivation is. Perhaps, at the end of the day, the couch and a box set beckons more than your exercise mat? However, if you ever needed a reason to start moving more, the recent pandemic was it! COVID-19 proved to be a mild illness for most, but for far too many, tragically, it was fatal. We have learnt the hard way about the importance of both being fit and a healthy weight. This did not guarantee survival, but it helped the odds. Many of us realised that we are not invincible, that we need to invest time now in our health to ensure we are fit enough to face any future challenges or illnesses.

Some elements of our lives are out of our control, yet others we can control. You can take steps to improve your health and wellbeing. How and when you exercise is within your control, so let's make sure you're doing it right.

> '*Physical activity is the first requisite of happiness. Our interpretation of physical fitness is the attainment and maintenance of a uniformly developed body with a sound mind fully capable of naturally, easily, and satisfactorily performing our many and varied daily tasks with spontaneous zest and pleasure.*'
>
> JOSEPH PILATES,
> —— *RETURN TO LIFE*

SIMPLY MOVE MORE – THE BENEFITS OF LITTLE & OFTEN

Unfortunately, only about 20 per cent of us are getting even a moderate level of regular exercise. And yet regular exercise, even walking, can reduce the risk of heart attack or stroke by a whopping 31 per cent. One study analysed 655,000 people and discovered that being active for a mere 11 minutes a day after the age of 40, added 1.8 years to life expectancy. If you exercise for an hour or more daily, that increases to an additional 4.2 years.

We are engineered to move not sit. Both the World Health Organization (WHO) and UK Chief Medical Officers identified that being sedentary has a profoundly negative effect on our health in their latest reports. Sitting has become the new smoking. We hope to show you how small bursts of exercise can be life changing, even life extending.

'Prolonged sitting is harmful, even in people who achieve the recommended levels of Moderate – Vigorous Physical Activity.'[1]

UK CHIEF MEDICAL OFFICERS

Recent research also demonstrated the benefits of taking regular breaks from sitting for people with type 2 diabetes – even brief breaks improved 24-hour glucose levels and insulin sensitivity.[2]

The more health-conscious amongst you may already set aside a couple of hours a week to 'exercise'. We certainly do not want you to stop coming to our Pilates classes! Nothing beats having a well-qualified teacher. However, the mini workouts show you how to make Pilates an integral part of your day. I treasure my two Pilates sessions with my teachers each week. They provide oases of calm between teaching, writing and grandmother duties. I am lucky that I do not have a desk job, but for those of you who work at a computer, how natural is it to sit at a desk all day and then 'exercise'?

Our ancestors didn't need to set aside 'exercise' time because their very survival involved vigorous activity all day, every day: hunting and gathering, building shelter, protecting family and territory. Our modern lives are very different. Now, all we hunt is the TV

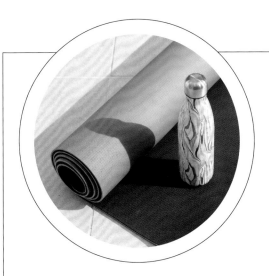

remote, and all we gather is that it was under the cushion where it always is! We are rarely challenged physically, unless through sport or exercise (or grandchildren). Even within my lifetime I have seen a dramatic change in daily activity. My grandmother used a mangle to dry the washing; a great workout for the arms. Shopping had to be carried as they never owned a car. I even remember having to help shovel coal into the coal bunker after school.

Combined with the advice on cardiovascular activities (pages 200–3) the Pilates Express® programme will substantially increase your overall levels of physical activity. One of the important changes to the advice in the most recent WHO report is that your aerobic activity no longer needs to be a minimum of 10 minutes to be beneficial:

'MVPA (Moderate – Vigorous Physical Activity) bouts of any duration now count towards these recommendations, reflecting new evidence to support the value of total physical activity volume, regardless of bout length.'[3]

WORLD HEALTH ORGANIZATION, 2020

While our workouts aim to tone and streamline, we also look at how to use exercise to get your immune and respiratory systems functioning well and explore ways to help you cope with stress better. Culminative chronic stress can influence your overall health and your weight. You will discover simple ways to reduce your stress levels and boost something called your Vagal Tone.

What is different about *Pilates Express*®?

HOW DOES THE PROGRAMME WORK?

If there is one message in this book it is that we need to view exercise not as a chore to tick off a list, but as part and parcel of our daily lives. There is potential for moving more and better in almost everything we do.

In every workout we are taking multi-tasking to the extreme. You will read the instruction 'simultaneously' with many of the exercise directions. We have created new exercises by applying our New Fundamentals and our Eight Principles (page 33). You'll also find variations of old favourites, which will challenge you in ways you cannot yet imagine. And we have cleverly combined exercises, not only to save time but to improve your co-ordination, movement, strength and flexibility.

For each exercise, we have identified specific challenges and benefits so that you are clear on what you are achieving. By challenging you physically we are encouraging your body to adapt, to become stronger, more mobile. Then if, in your daily activities, you need to reach and lift and twist, your body has the mobility and strength to manage it, with ease and without strain.

We have designed around 40 10-minute workouts for you to intersperse through your day, at work or at home. Each one is balanced and will get your muscles pumping, stimulating your lymphatic system while reminding you of good posture. By mobilising joints, we work on flexibility, by using the body's own weight against gravity, we tone your whole body. Our controlled breathing practices will help your mood, lifting your spirits. Rather than doing a wide range of exercises in each workout, we focus on doing a few really well. **Every breath, every movement counts.** We want your 10-minute workouts to have an impact on how you feel, look, think and move for the remainder of the day.

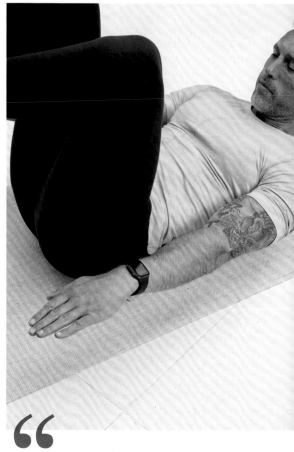

'Something old, something new, something borrowed, something to stop you being blue...'

The Pilates Express® Day

Whenever you can, exercise outdoors (see page 185). If you can find level ground, you can do the mat-based exercises, otherwise we've also given you lots of Standing Workouts.

MORNING WORKOUTS

These exercises stretch you out after sleep and energise you. Your posture will be set for the day. You'll leave the house taller, more supple, breathing better, your mind focused, ready to face the day's challenges. Most morning workouts will be mat-based, but you'll find some Standing Workouts too.

MIDDAY WORKOUTS

Choose between Seated, Standing and Sit to Stand, Stand to Sit Workouts. Ideally, you would do the Standing Workouts, even better you would do them outside, in a forest. But we know that not everyone can leave their desks, so we've given you options.

The **Seated Workouts** will move your spine in every direction. It is very easy to forget good posture when you're at work. If you are working from home, it can be worse still with some of us working on computers at the dining table, in armchairs or, heaven forbid, from bed. Your spine is compressed, the vertebrae may twist unnaturally, your neck strains. It is no wonder you may be experiencing backache and tension headaches! It can even impact your sleep as the change to your neck angle affects the joint that connects your jawbone and skull. This can change the position of your teeth, causing bruxism, or teeth grinding. Our 10-minute fixes will remind you of good posture, moving those joints which stiffen when you sit for too long. The breathing exercises will rejuvenate and calm you. The immunity exercises will keep your lymph flowing. Your afternoons will become as productive as your mornings! The **Standing Workouts** are great to do anywhere.

Then, for the first time, we are introducing the **Sit to Stand, Stand to Sit (STS) Workouts**. A study conducted in March 2015 found that, on average, most of us complete the STS manoeuvre at least 45 times a day![4] We give you instructions on how to STS better, so that your muscles are balanced, joints aligned. The STS workouts contain a mix of sitting, standing and STS manoeuvres.

EVENING WORKOUTS

We've given you a choice, depending on how you are feeling. You can choose a Strength and Flexibility Workout that will tone you top to toe. Or you can do a Relaxing Workout to iron out any kinks in your spine, and calm both mind and body. We have also given the option of a Mindful Pilates session at any time instead of, or as well as, your mini workout.

Before you do anything, however, go to the New Fundamentals chapter. If you are new to Pilates, you will learn the basics. If you are a veteran, you can update yourself on the latest approach. Alignment, Breathing and Centring are the ABCs of our approach. The Alignment section shows you how to position yourself correctly in the Starting Positions. There are traditional Starting Positions and some newcomers, such as Lunges and Split Stance. You need to learn how to control your Alignment through movement too. We introduce you to your Centreline, which is very useful for checking Alignment. You will then move on to efficient Breathing. In this section, you'll encounter not just Pilates-style lateral thoracic breathing but also new approaches. Then, we have dedicated a chapter to Respiratory Health (page 54) to help you assess your breathing pattern and explore techniques to improve its efficiency. The final section of The New Fundamentals is dedicated to Centring – how to engage your deep core muscles and use them appropriately while exercising.

Next, try the Exercises for Respiratory Health (pages 94–121). If you can improve your breathing, you'll get so much more out of the workouts (and life). You can then move on to Exercises for Immune Health (pages 122–153). And, when you're ready for a greater challenge, try the Strength and Flexibility exercises (pages 154–177). When you feel you have learnt the exercises, you're ready for the Workouts, where you'll find exercises drawn from all these chapters. If you manage to do just one workout a day, by the end of the week you will have done the equivalent of a 70-minute workout.

Joseph Pilates' Legacy on Health

> ❝
>
> *'Only through the attainment of perfect balance of mind and body, can one appreciate what really constitutes normal health.'*
>
> JOSEPH PILATES,
> —— *RETURN TO LIFE*

But first a word about our founder and his approach to health, because Joseph Pilates had a lot to say about lifestyle. He wrote *Your Health* and *Return to Life through Contrology* in 1934 and 1945 respectively and always believed that his exercise method was ahead of its time. When he died in 1967, Contrology was still a very niche form of exercise. It has taken decades for the world to catch up.

When you read his books, you realise how much sound lifestyle advice there is which is now being reinforced by research. Not every part of Joe's teaching was correct. He believed our spines should be ramrod straight, for example, that we should sleep in V-shaped beds and that masturbation was the 'curse of mankind'! But his emphasis on mental, as well as physical, health has never been more relevant.

Joe also believed in the benefits of fresh air and sunlight, and exposure to cold. He advocates minimal clothing, which he believed helped make us more resilient. Many of the photographs we have of him show him outside in his underwear. He writes that our bodies also 'breathe' through the pores of the skin. In one photo, he is nearly 80 and standing in snow in the Catskill Mountains wearing just underpants and soft-soled shoes! In his New York studio, clients were encouraged to shower after class and use a stiff brush to exfoliate and massage their limbs. He was rumoured to have hopped in with you if he felt you weren't using the stiff brush firmly enough!

While he did not write at length about nutrition, he did urge moderation: 'The principal point to remember, with regards to diet, is to eat only enough food to restore the "fuel" consumed by the body...' Not only did he understand the importance of sleep, he also recognised what helped us sleep well: 'Most important, in the matter of enjoying good recuperative sleep are quiet, darkness, fresh air and mental calm.'

Joe also placed relaxation and socialising with friends and family high on his list of activities for good health, encouraging us to embrace 'every possible form of pleasurable living. For example, simply spending a quiet and pleasant evening at home with family chatting with congenial friends, is accordingly to our interpretation, a form of play that is delightful, pleasant social entertainment.'

Above all, he wanted us to understand the connection between mind and body. Correct posture, breathing and uniform development of muscles are the key: 'Contrology develops the body uniformly, corrects wrong postures, restores physical vitality, invigorates the mind, and elevates the spirit.'

I do not think Joe would have been at all surprised about the growing popularity of his method today. He knew it worked. People all over the world are benefiting from his work.

The Benefits of Pilates

Here are some benefits of regular Pilates that our clients report:

1. IMPROVED BODY AWARENESS

2. BETTER POSTURE

3. INCREASED SPINE FLEXIBILITY AND STRENGTH

4. IMPROVED JOINT MOBILITY, RESULTING IN FEWER JOINT ACHES AND PAINS

5. IMPROVED BALANCE AND CO-ORDINATION

6. MORE EFFICIENT BREATHING

7. IMPROVED BONE STRENGTH

8. INCREASED STAMINA AND ENERGY

9. STRONGER MUSCLES; IN PARTICULAR THE GLUTEALS, QUADRICEPS, HAMSTRINGS, CALVES, UPPER ARMS, BACK AND ABDOMINALS AND PELVIC FLOOR.

10. A MORE STREAMLINED OUTLINE, ESPECIALLY A TRIMMER WAISTLINE

11. HEALTHIER, LESS PAINFUL FEET

12. IMPROVED SLEEP

13. IMPROVED SELF-ESTEEM AND CONFIDENCE

14. HELP MANAGING CONDITIONS OF THE MIND AND EMOTIONS; THE MINDFULNESS OF PILATES IS VERY BENEFICIAL TO MENTAL AS WELL AS PHYSICAL HEALTH

15. A FEELING OF GENERAL HEALTH AND WELLBEING

16. BETTER ABILITY TO COPE WITH STRESS

17. BALANCES YOUR BODY

Your Weight
——*The Dangers of Being Overweight*

We come in various shapes and sizes, and should celebrate this diversity, but there is no escaping the fact that being overweight carries serious health risks. A recent study of over 500,000 people revealed that we cannot be both overweight and healthy.[5] 'One cannot be fat but healthy,' writes Dr Lucia. 'Our findings refute the notion that a physically active lifestyle can completely negate the deleterious effects of overweight and obesity.' While regular exercise reduces the risk of developing health problems, such as high blood pressure and diabetes, if you are overweight you're still at risk of heart attacks and strokes.

The recent pandemic also reconfirmed the link between good health and weight. Sadly, being obese seemed to worsen the effects of COVID-19. The Centers for Disease Control and Prevention (CDC) reported that people with heart disease and diabetes, both obesity-related conditions, are at higher risk of developing complications. Public Health England also found that excess weight put people at greater risk of needing hospital admission or intensive care. The risk grows as weight increases. If you ever needed motivation to lose weight, this was it!

Obesity reduces life expectancy by an average of 3–10 years, depending on how severe it is. It is estimated that obesity and being overweight contribute to at least one in every 13 deaths in Europe.

"

'Fighting obesity and inactivity is equally important, it should be a joint battle.'

DR ALEJANDRO LUCIA
—— *MD, PhD University of Madrid, Centre for Research in Sport and Physical Activity*

The risks associated with being overweight are serious and many.

THEY INCLUDE:

• Type 2 diabetes

• High blood pressure

• High cholesterol and atherosclerosis (where fatty deposits narrow your arteries), which can lead to coronary heart disease and stroke

• Asthma

• Metabolic syndrome (a combination of diabetes, high blood pressure and obesity)

• Several types of cancer, including bowel, breast and womb

• Gastro-oesophageal reflux disease (GORD) (where stomach acid leaks out of the stomach and into the gullet)

• Gallstones

• Reduced fertility

• Osteoarthritis (a condition involving pain and stiffness in your joints)

• Sleep apnoea (a condition that causes interrupted breathing during sleep, which can lead to daytime sleepiness with an increased risk of road traffic accidents, as well as a greater risk of diabetes, high blood pressure and heart disease)

• Liver disease and kidney disease

• Pregnancy complications, such as gestational diabetes or pre-eclampsia (when a woman experiences a potentially dangerous rise in blood pressure during pregnancy)

The Waist to Height Ratio Check

The easiest way to check if you need to lose weight is the Waist to Height ratio check. This is far simpler than calculating your Body Mass Index, which can give a false reading. It will also give you an idea if you are carrying extra weight around your middle, which means you may have visceral fat around your internal organs, liver, kidneys and heart. This fat may have started to produce hormones and chemicals which increase your risk of obesity-related diseases.

Take a piece of string and use it to measure your height. Fold the string in half and place it around your waist, level with your navel.

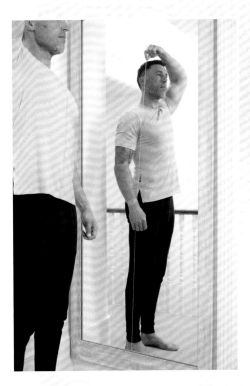

- If the halved string does not reach around your waist, you are carrying too much weight around your middle. Ideally, your waist circumference should be 50 per cent of your height measurement.

- But if your waist is 60–70 per cent you would be considered overweight and that carries extra risk.

- If your waist measures over 70 per cent, you would be considered obese, which carries even more risk.

- Over 80 per cent and you are classed as morbidly obese, which further increases all the risks.

Losing Weight – A Complex Issue

According to the WHO, the fundamental cause of obesity is the energy imbalance between calories consumed and calories expended. Worldwide, in recent years, we have seen:

- An increased intake of energy-dense foods that are high in fat.

- An increase in physical inactivity due to the increasingly sedentary nature of many forms of work, changing modes of transportation and increasing urbanisation.

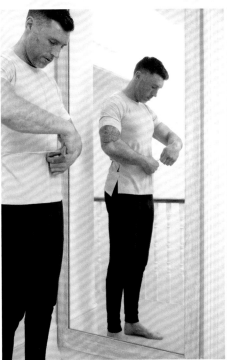

Increased portion size has been blamed and, it seems, we are putting more of the wrong type of food on our plates. It is not just the equation of eat less, move more: many other factors influence weight. Genetics play a role, getting enough sunshine and darkness, sleeping well and managing stress. In the next chapter, we'll look at how long-term stress affects wellbeing. Chronic stress can also cause metabolic changes that lead to weight gain. It interferes with your hunger and satiety (feeling full) messengers, making you crave certain foods (usually fatty, salty, sugary ones!). Stress 'convinces' your body that it is in times of hardship; better eat more.

Chronic Stress ——
The Enemy of Good Physical and Mental Health

It is strange to think that the word 'stress', used with its current meaning, was first coined by Hans Selye just 50 years ago! Selye identified that it is not stress itself that causes health problems, but how we respond to it, or to be more precise, how we recover from a stressful situation.

FIGHT OR FLIGHT VS REST & DIGEST

To understand this better, we need to discuss the 'fight or flight' response, so named because our ancestors, when faced with danger, had to choose between fighting or fleeing. Thankfully, there are not many woolly mammoths and sabre-toothed tigers around today for us to contend with, but you only have to open a newspaper to read about modern dangers, such as violent crime, car accidents, terrorist attacks and natural disasters. The recent COVID-19 pandemic was life-threatening and many of us are still recovering from its impact.

In addition, we all face less life-threatening stresses daily, such as money troubles, approaching work deadlines, marital stress and examinations. In *Can't Even: How Millennials Became the Burnout Generation* Anne Helen Petersen explores the reasons behind the total exhaustion felt by many born between 1981–1996. She identifies the common feeling of constantly falling short, a perceived sense of failure, financial instability and the fear of wasting time as culprits. Even during leisure hours, millennials feel the need to be productive – they have lost the art of doing nothing.

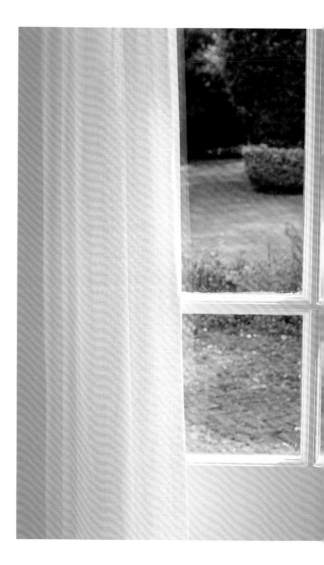

No wonder Millenials feel under pressue. Chronic stress may not always be the cause of the problem, of course, but it can be a contributing factor.

When confronting what you perceive as a threat, your autonomic nervous system takes over. (Autonomic means a process that works without having to think about it.) This system is divided into two channels: sympathetic and parasympathetic nervous systems.

The sympathetic nervous system signals activation of your flight or fight response. Adrenaline and cortisol, the stress hormone, are released. Once released, they affect your heart rate. Your heart beats faster to bring oxygen to major muscles, which you need to either run or do battle. Your breathing speeds up to deliver more oxygen to your blood. Your peripheral vision increases (in case danger approaches from the side or behind). Your pupils dilate to allow you to see better. Your hearing sharpens. You may sweat more or get goosebumps. Your hands and feet might feel cold as blood is redirected to major muscles to prepare for action. Digestion of any food may be interrupted, and you may feel sick, vomit, or involuntarily relieve yourself. Your perception of pain might be temporarily reduced as survival becomes a priority.

If the 'danger' resulted in an injury or infection, the area may become inflamed to start the healing process. Inflammation of an injured area, or in response to a virus or infection, is an essential part of healing. Blood vessels dilate to increase blood flow, bringing white blood cells to fight off 'invaders'. Swelling puts pressure on nerves and makes the area tender. These white blood cells discharge chemicals called cytokines. These cytokines can cause you to feel feverish, but are, in fact, vital in the fight against infection. However, health problems arise if your body overreacts

> *'It is not the stress that kills us...it's our reaction to it.'*
>
> HANS SELYE, ——————
> PIONEERING HUNGARIAN-CANADIAN
> ENDOCRINOLOGIST

to an infection (cytokine storm), underreacts, or if the inflammation remains in the body long term. Chronic inflammation is the cause of many degenerative diseases.

Overreacting can be fatal. One of the causes of fatalities from COVID-19 was victims' immune systems 'over responding' to the virus, causing a cytokine storm. This created high levels of inflammation throughout their bodies.

The sympathetic nervous system is not only activated when you are threatened. It kicks in when you are faced with stressful events, such as the first day back at school, a job interview, public speaking or a sports match. Normally, when the 'danger' (infection, virus, injury, stressful event) has passed, the parasympathetic nervous system takes over to counterbalance the sympathetic nervous system by calming and relaxing your body, allowing you to 'rest and digest' again. Your heart rate and breathing slow, your blood pressure lowers and any inflammation starts to reduce. You are 'safe'.

Central to this balancing act between the parasympathetic and sympathetic nervous systems is the vagus nerve, the longest nerve of your autonomic, parasympathetic nervous system. It is responsible for regulating your heart rate, slowing your pulse and turning organs on and off in response to stress. It connects your brain and vital organs, including the stomach, lungs, heart, spleen, liver and kidneys. It keeps you healthy by regulating the immune system, controlling stress levels and reducing inflammation. It also plays a key role in preventing the immune system from overreacting and over-responding.

The Polyvagal Theory —— *Fight, Flight or Freeze*

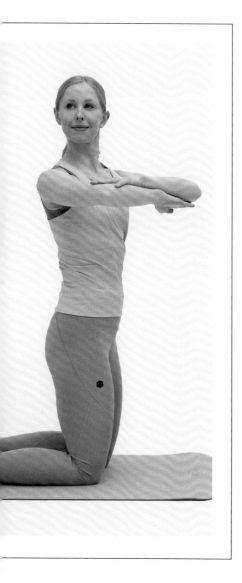

The vagus nerve has been the subject of a lot of recent research largely due to the ground-breaking work of Dr Stephen Porges, Professor of Psychiatry at the University of North Carolina. In *The Polyvagal Theory*, he writes that in response to danger, your body may prepare to fight or flee, or it may 'freeze', that is, become immobilised with fear. This can result in you being rooted to the spot, or even fainting. You see this in the animal kingdom, where animals play dead to escape predators.

The Polyvagal theory emphasises that your nervous system has more than one defence strategy and that the decision to fight, flee or freeze is not something you can control. He also discovered that, contrary to previous beliefs, the parasympathetic system has two branches: a ventral vagal complex (VVC) and a dorsal vagal complex (DVC). These branches lead to different physiological states, hence the name 'polyvagal theory'. The VVC concerns itself with the nerves at the front and top part of the chest, above the diaphragm, connecting the facial muscles of expression and hearing, with the heart. This complex contributes to social behaviour. We smile if we are friendly, scowl or growl if not. If you are on the receiving end of friendly signals, it can tell you that you are in a safe environment. As a result, your heart rate relaxes, breathing slows. This regular social interaction with friends, family and community keeps us healthy. No wonder that national lockdowns during the pandemic had such a devastating effect on people isolating alone.

Meanwhile, the DVC, the more primeval of the two channels, serves nerves to structures below the diaphragm, especially your digestive system. Its activation can lead to a 'shutdown' and withdrawal, accompanied by lethargy, a lowered heart rate and potential digestive problems, like Irritable Bowel Syndrome.

The Polyvagal theory has revolutionised the treatment of many mental health issues; amongst other things, post-traumatic stress disorder. Dr Porges explains that your nervous system can affect your behaviour, based on how safe or how threatened you feel. Surrounding yourself with warmth, smiles and laughter and affirmative messages helps you heal.

The Importance of Good Vagal Tone

How well you cope with stress depends on your 'vagal tone', which is an indicator of how well your vagal subsystems are working. Some people have better vagal tone than others: those with good vagal tone find it easier to relax after a stressful period. Others, with weaker vagal tone, find it harder to de-stress. The difference in individual vagal tone is known as Heart Rate Variability or HRV (the vagus nerve regulates heart rate). Measuring your HRV can give an indication of how well you cope with stress.

Poor vagal tone has been linked with some chronic inflammatory diseases.[6] In 2013, researchers discovered a positive feedback loop between high vagal tone and good physical health. The more you increase your vagal tone, the more your physical and mental health will improve and vice versa. To some degree, you inherit good or poor vagal tone from your parents, but that does not mean you cannot do something about it. We have already seen that being around positive, happy, loving family and friends is enormously beneficial. There are also other things you can do. Jordan Fallis, Founder and CEO of Optimal Living Dynamics, in his article 'How to Stimulate Your Vagus Nerve for Better Mental Health', lists nine ways to improve vagal tone:

1. **COLD EXPOSURE**
2. **SINGING, HUMMING, CHANTING AND GARGLING**
3. **PROBIOTICS**
4. **OMEGA-3 FATTY ACIDS**
5. **MASSAGE**
6. **SOCIALISING AND LAUGHING**
7. **EXERCISE**
8. **MEDITATION AND MINDFULNESS**
9. **DEEP AND SLOW BREATHING**

When I read this article, I was blown away by the similarities between Fallis' advice and that found in Joseph Pilates' two books. Compare this list to the one on page 8 and you will see that Joseph Pilates advocated many of the same activities, nearly 80 years before the above article was published!

Note: Spending time with pets is another recommended way to improve vagal tone. Pets can provide comfort and companionship. Personally, I find it incredibly calming, and reassuring, when one of my cats jumps on my lap for a stroke. Maybe slightly less relaxing when they walk over my keyboard or if I'm chasing 'dead' mice!

The 9-Point Plan *to Improve Vagal Tone*

Note that I have changed the order of Fallis' plan.

1. COLD EXPOSURE

We know this is something Joseph Pilates believed in. But if rolling in the snow in your underwear seems too daunting, a cold blast of the shower will suffice. Or a trip to a sauna, followed by an ice bath. Wild swimming is becoming increasingly popular. Ensure you join a local wild swimming club as there are dangers in swimming in lakes and rivers. Visit www.wildswimming.co.uk or www.outdoorswimmingsociety.com for advice.

2. SINGING, HUMMING, CHANTING & GARGLING

Unfortunately, I am not sure I would have any clients left if I started singing in my classes. Instead, I reserve my efforts for when I'm alone or with the grandchildren, who, bless them, don't seem to mind. But we can all recognise the joy of singing, whether alone or in a group, whether you are in tune or tone deaf. It is hard to be sad while singing (Leonard Cohen may have been the exception). And, of course, when you are singing you are also controlling your breathing (see below).

Humming is a habit I have always had, much to the annoyance of my husband. Strangely, or maybe not on reflection, I can remember my dear father humming whenever he had to reverse park the car, which he found tricky. Perhaps, intuitively, he knew it relaxed him.

It might be a good idea to hum for a few minutes before you try some of the breathing exercises.

Research has shown humming helps to clear your sinuses by creating turbulence in the air which, when we exhale, helps move air and mucus out more forcefully than normal quiet breathing.[7]

Chanting has been used in most religions for centuries, from Gregorian chants to Buddhist Om chanting. Advocates claim many health benefits, including improved concentration, reduced stress and anxiety, detoxification of the body, improved heart and digestive function, and sound sleep.

Gargling and salt water rinsing are age-old remedies credited with many health benefits, including helping sinus infections, as well as sore throats, colds, flu, allergies and oral health. If you wish to try gargling, mix ½ teaspoon of salt with 225ml (8 fl oz) warm water. Do not swallow the water, spit it out. (Always check with your doctor before you try gargling for a medical condition.) Amazingly, while I was researching for this book, I discovered a paragraph in Joseph Pilates' *Your Health* advocating neti, the ancient practice of rinsing the sinuses with salt water.

3. PROBIOTICS

Taking a good probiotic is straightforward and there are lots of excellent products available. But as Helen Ford, our nutritionist in *Shape Up with Pilates*, pointed out, you can find these bacteria in yogurt (plain yogurt is best as fruit yogurt can contain a lot of added sugar). Fermented foods such as miso and natto, kimchi, sauerkraut and kefir are examples from around the world. (More about probiotics on page 27.)

4. OMEGA-3 FATTY ACIDS

Omega-3 is an essential fat, so called because we cannot manufacture it within our bodies and it's essential for pretty much every cell. Found predominantly in oily fish (tinned is an excellent source and sometimes better than fresh), walnuts, chia seeds, hemp and flaxseed. High blood sugar has been linked to low levels of omega-3 because cells become resistant to insulin, which is a major factor in weight gain and type 2 diabetes.

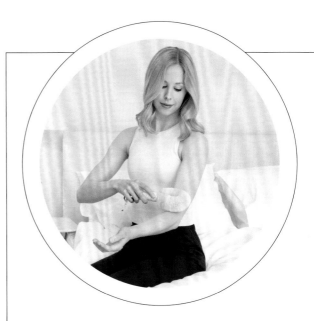

5. MASSAGE

There are many types of massage to choose from, some pampering and indulgent, others more medical and therapeutic (though you could argue that all massage is therapeutic). First, decide what you want the massage to focus on, for example muscular pain, deep tissue, fascia release, lymphatic drainage. Then, search for an appropriately qualified therapist, who is registered with a recognised professional body, such as The General Council for Soft Tissue Therapies, The Association for Soft Tissue Therapists – the SMA, or the National Association of Massage and Manipulative Therapists.

It is not easy to self-massage, so you could also try skin brushing, as recommended by Joseph Pilates. Skin brushing stimulates both the circulation of blood and the lymphatic system, helping to eliminate toxins and waste products. To get the best results, brush the skin when it is dry using a natural fibre body brush with firm bristles. Start gently, using light strokes and increase the pressure over the first week. Morning is the best time to kick-start your day, but after exercise, as Joe recommended, is also beneficial.

- The golden rule is always stroke towards your heart, encouraging rather than fighting the flow of your body's natural systems.

- Making sure you are steady, brush the sole of each foot in turn.

- Work up your lower legs, then from the knee to pelvic bone using long sweeping movements. With each stroke, use your free hand to follow the brush, soothing the skin.

- Continue over your buttocks and hips, then switch to circular clockwise strokes over your stomach.

- Move on to your arms, starting at the fingertips and sweeping towards your chest, along your shoulders and down your breastbone to the heart.

- Reach around your back and stroke down each side. If your brush has a long handle, you should be able to reach your middle back too.

6. SOCIALISING & LAUGHING

Smile more! Laugh more! I am always telling new Pilates teachers that, while it is very important to ensure good Pilates technique in classes, it is equally important to have a good laugh. Apart from anything else, it works the transversus, one of your deep core muscles. Sometimes, us Pilates teachers take ourselves too seriously, especially with regards to giving corrections. Yes, we have given you lists of Watchpoints for how to perform the exercises in this book correctly, but please don't worry if you find them difficult. It is a cliché, but practice makes perfect and, in the meantime, every movement and every smile helps.
Dr Stephen Porges emphasised the importance of surrounding ourselves with friendly faces. Once again, Joseph Pilates also believed in the value of relaxing with and 'chatting with congenial friends' (page 8).

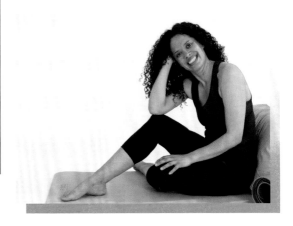

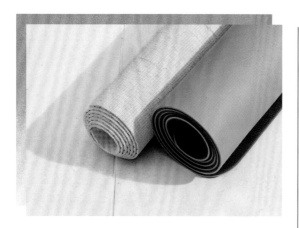

7. EXERCISE

If you need any more motivation to move, regular physical activity comes with a fine list of benefits. Movement and exercise improve your immune system function (page 24) by increasing the activity of 'natural killer cells', the immune cells that kill infection. They also promote the creation of new mitochondria, which in turn enhances your ability to create energy. They help to reduce inflammation, improve blood pressure and circulatory and lymphatic flow (page 25). They change your gut microbiota and regulate hormonal dysfunction. Are you sold yet? If not, movement and exercise, even just walking regularly, may help prevent Alzheimer's. Regular exercise reduces the risk of cancer, heart attacks, strokes and lessens your risk of developing type 2 diabetes.

Working on muscle strength means your body releases the chemical messengers cytokines (page 13). One of these cytokines, interleukin, plays a crucial role in switching off the inflammation process. As we age, good muscle strength also means a reduced risk of osteoporosis. And one of the reasons why you feel great after exercise is because it releases endorphins, the feel-good hormones.

8. MEDITATION & MINDFULNESS

Meditation is the process of training your mind to focus and redirect your thoughts. It is a practice that yields many health benefits. Studies show it may improve symptoms of stress-related conditions, such as irritable bowel syndrome (IBS)[8], PTSD[9] and fibromyalgia[10]. It can help with the management of chronic pain, improve symptoms of depression and reduce anxiety. It may also reduce age-related memory loss. It can also help in the fight against addictions and aid sleep as well as lowering blood pressure.[11] It is starting to look like meditation is another 'miracle cure' we can use alongside exercise! For more information on meditation, see page 204.

If you find meditation difficult, as I do, you might like to try a mindfulness exercise instead. This can be particularly helpful if you suffer from 'monkey mind' and find it hard to concentrate during meditation. Mindfulness is not meditation as it is a quality, rather than a practice. However, it is part of the meditation process. Like meditation, mindfulness can be defined as focusing fully on your current experience and is the opposite of automatic pilot (where your mind just wanders). Mindfulness is about being fully present and experiencing the world firmly in the 'here and now'. It is also about being non-judgemental. Its benefits are wide reaching; for example, it has been used with mental health problems, helping to ease anxiety and mental stress.[12]

As this is a book which is encouraging you to move more throughout your day, applying mindfulness to movement may be more appropriate. In truth, all your Pilates practice should be done mindfully. You should be fully focused on your breathing, alignment and movements but you can increase this level of awareness. On page 198 you will find one example of the Mindful Pilates approach applied to Spine Curls. (I hope we can write a book on Mindful Pilates in the near future – watch this space.) You can practise mindfulness at any time, but morning is particularly beneficial as it clears your mind and prepares you for the day. It's a good idea to substitute a Mindful Pilates session for one of your mini workouts. Or, even better, as well as your Morning, Midday or Evening Workout.

9. DEEP, SLOW, CONTROLLED BREATHING

This requires a whole chapter.

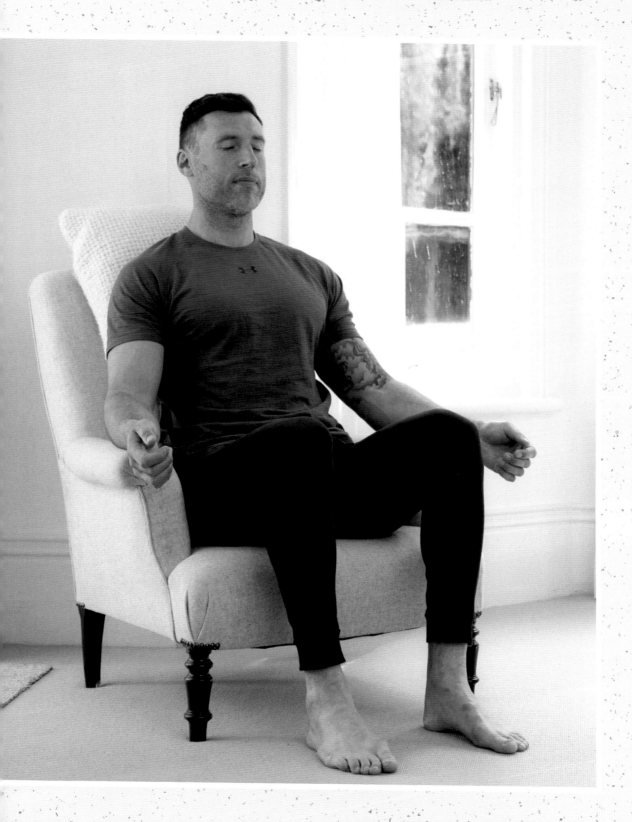

Controlled Breathing *to Improve Vagal Tone*

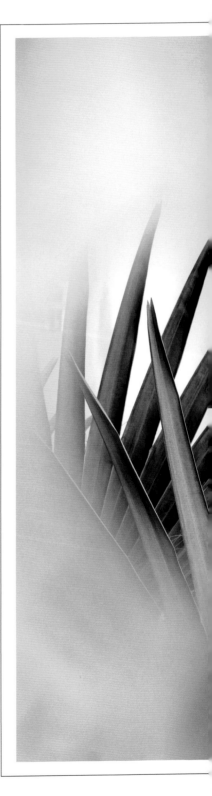

Next time you are anxious or stressed, notice how you are breathing. Then compare the rate of your breathing to how you breathe when you are relaxed. When you are stressed, your breathing rate becomes 'apical' – you take small, shallow breaths, you may even hyperventilate. You end up using your shoulders and upper chest more, rather than your diaphragm. This is not a problem short term, but if you carry on breathing this way, it can upset the balance of gases in the body and may make you feel anxious and stressed. Thankfully, numerous studies show how controlled breathing practices can calm you.[13]

Breathing is an autonomic function. You can control it for short periods, but ultimate control rests with your brain, where receptors regulate the rate and volume of breathing. However, you can, as we do in the exercise programme, use quiet, slow and rhythmic, controlled breathing, to help calm the nervous system that controls involuntary functions. When you breathe in, the heart speeds the flow of oxygenated blood throughout the body via your arteries, and as you breathe out your heart rate slows. In this way, you can stimulate the vagus nerve and improve vagal tone with exercises involving deep, controlled breathing. If you can slow your breathing, breathe deeply, but gently, evenly and rhythmically, you can 'open up' communication along the vagal network and relax yourself into a parasympathetic state. Basically, our breathing exercises can tell your body that the danger has passed.

The best type of breathing to help vagal tone involves making your exhalation longer than your inhalation. Later in the book, we share breathing exercises for better vagal tone. The most common breathing pattern used in Pilates involves a longer exhalation. The general rule for most, if not all, exercises is to ...

- Breathe in to prepare for movement.
- Breathe out as you perform the movement.
- Breathe in, either on the return, or take an extra in breath and return on the exhale.

If you time yourself doing an exercise such as Roll Downs, Ribcage Closure or Spine Curls, you will discover that your exhalation is likely to be longer than your inhalation.

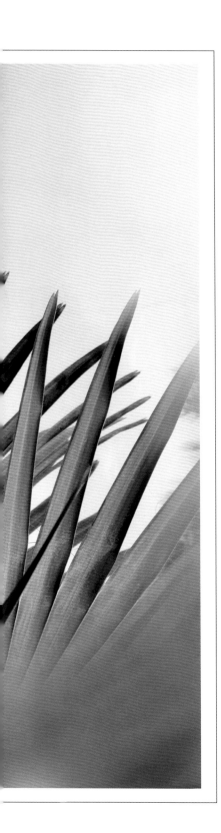

Controlled Movement & Stress Levels

Anyone who practises Pilates regularly will testify to the profound influence it has on mental wellbeing. I find there is a magical moment, usually about ten minutes into a class, when worries fall away and the world seems a better place. This may be linked to the controlled breathing and its impact on vagal tone, or the fact that I'm so focused on controlling my limbs that I cannot think about anything else! But there is another theory. Research from the University of Pittsburgh, published in *The Proceedings of the National Academy of Sciences of the USA*, gave a fresh insight into why Pilates (and other mind–body practices like yoga and t'ai chi) leave us feeling free from stress. The research provided evidence for the neural basis of the mind–body connection. They discovered a circuit that directly links the cerebral cortex (part of the brain) to the adrenal medulla. The adrenal medulla is the inner part of the adrenal gland responsible for your flight, fight or freeze response to stressful situations. The adrenal medulla triggers the adrenal surge when you are faced with danger. And, and this is the best bit, it seems that this very same brain network is also associated with the motor cortex, which controls movements.

'One of these areas is a portion of the primary motor cortex that is concerned with the control of axial body movement and posture. This input to the adrenal medulla may explain why core body exercises are so helpful in modulating responses to stress.'

It may not just be the controlled breathing, but also the controlled movements of Pilates that help regulate stress. In the New Fundamentals chapter, we introduce you to your Centreline. Many of the exercises in this programme ask you to be aware of your Centreline and move through it and around it, thus promoting control of your 'axial body movement and posture'.

But let us look now at how important it is to learn how to breathe well.

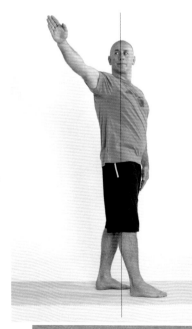

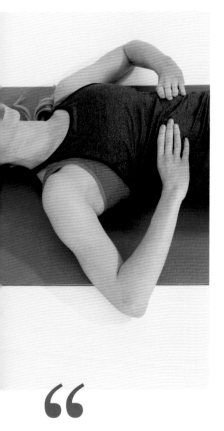

"

'... the first lesson is that of correct breathing.'

JOSEPH PILATES,
—————— *YOUR HEALTH*

Your Respiratory Health

Joseph Pilates was acutely aware of why good breathing matters. As a child, he suffered with asthma and, in later life, from emphysema, aggravated by smoke inhalation from a fire in his studio and probably not helped by his love of cigars! That he lived to nearly 80, and was incredibly active until the very end, is testament to the effectiveness of his exercise method. He pleaded with the US government to adopt 'Contrology' to help in the fight against tuberculosis.

Learning to breathe better will transform your health. We have lots of breathwork in this book, but first, let's look at the process of breathing as this will help you understand how best to improve it.

THE PROCESS OF RESPIRATION

'Respiration' is not the same as breathing, which is properly called 'ventilation'. Respiration is the chemical reaction that happens in all your cells. All cells need oxygen to create energy efficiently. When they create energy, they make carbon dioxide. When you breathe in, oxygen comes into your body and travels via the trachea to your lungs. The oxygen is absorbed through capillaries in the lungs and enters the blood to be pumped throughout the body by your heart. Every cell absorbs oxygen, after which the deoxygenated blood, carbon dioxide and 'waste products' are transported back to the lungs by your veins. The carbon dioxide is expelled as you breathe out. When carbon dioxide reaches a certain level, a signal is sent from your brain to your breathing muscles, which triggers inhalation. The more active you are, the more carbon dioxide is produced, which is why you breathe more when physically active. However, we should not think of carbon dioxide as a waste product, explains Patrick McKeown in *The Oxygen Advantage*:

'It is a key variable that allows the release of oxygen from the red blood cells to be metabolized by the body .... When we breathe correctly, we have sufficient amount of carbon dioxide, and our breathing is quiet, controlled and rhythmic.'

Carbon dioxide forces oxygen to leave the blood so that it can enter your muscles and organs. This is called the Bohr effect, named after Christian Bohr, the Danish scientist who discovered its importance in 1904. Carbon dioxide also plays a role in other vital functions, such as widening and relaxing your smooth muscles (situated in your stomach, intestines, bladder, womb) and, also, in the regulation of your blood pH.

ARE YOU OVER-BREATHING?

Instead of the normal 8–12 breaths, many of us are taking 18–25 breaths per minute. This can upset the delicate balance between oxygen and carbon dioxide levels. As a result, your muscles do not work as effectively as they should. Habitual over-breathing can influence the release of oxygen from red blood cells, causing the narrowing of airways, limiting your body's ability to oxygenate and constricting blood vessels, reducing blood flow to the heart and other organs and muscles. This can impact your wellbeing, writes McKeown, who cites cardiovascular, respiratory and gastrointestinal issues, alongside anxiety, insomnia, exhaustion and even obesity as possible side effects. In the breathing exercises (pages 54-57), we encourage you to breathe in a 'quiet, controlled and rhythmic way'. We are aiming to regulate your breathing, and the starting point is to breathe both in and out through your nose, not mouth.

THE IMPORTANCE OF NASAL BREATHING

Nasal breathing is not just the most efficient way of breathing, you can argue that it is also what nature intended. The tiny hairs inside your nose filter pollutants, germs and bacteria from the air as you breathe in. The air is also warmed and humified, which means it is better received by your lungs. Nasal breathing results in 10–20 per cent more oxygen intake. It may take practice, especially if you have blocked sinuses, but it is well worth the effort.

BREATHING, POSTURE & STABILITY

There are many muscles involved in breathing, some more with inhalation, some with exhalation, some with both. The primary muscle is the diaphragm; a large, dome-shaped muscle which flattens as it contracts, on the inhale, allowing the lungs to expand. The muscles between the ribs also contract and pull upward, increasing the thoracic cavity and decreasing pressure inside. As a result, air rushes in and fills the lungs. As you exhale, the diaphragm relaxes, the volume inside the thoracic cavity decreases, while the pressure inside increases. The lungs therefore contract and air is forced out.

There is a strong connection between posture and breathing. The diaphragm is a key player in core stability, along with your abdominals and pelvic floor. It is part of the group of muscles that create the inner cylinder of intra-abdominal pressure, which stabilises your trunk[14] (Centring, page 58). However, the diaphragm's primary task will always be to facilitate breathing. If there is an increase in respiratory demand, for example during heavy cardiovascular work, the diaphragm prioritises respiration and your trunk stability may have to rely on other muscles.[15] This is why we want you to master The New Fundamentals. By breathing efficiently and connecting appropriately to your core, you encourage the right balance of oxygen and carbon dioxide, and the right muscles doing the right work. Remember too, that poor posture will impact your ability to breathe well. Slouching inhibits your transversus abdominis and pelvic floor muscles from working properly and stops the diaphragm descending properly during inhalation. We encourage you to stand, sit and walk tall, opening your chest, creating space internally for your ribcage to expand and for you to breathe.

THE FLEXIBLE RIBCAGE

The Exercises for Respiratory Health encourage the flexibility of your upper spine and ribcage. The ribcage consists of more than 80 joints and, while it has a protective role, it should not be considered a fixed structure, but a flexible, pliable cage. The more mobility in your upper spine and ribs, the better your ability to breathe! Spinal rotation exercises (twisting) are particularly good for mobilising your upper body. Exercises such as Bow and Arrow (page 86), Waist Twists (page 85), Hip Rolls with Rib Rolls (page 110), Threading the Needle (page 112) and all their variations all help. Then you can use spinal lateral flexion (side bending) exercises to open and expand the sides of your ribcage. Exercises such as Side Reach (page 89), Side Stretch (page 102) and Mermaid (page 117). Mobilising your upper spine into flexion and extension is also helpful. Exercises like Cat (page 80), Cobra Prep (page 168) and Curl Ups (page 84). Challenge yourself with combinations such as Mermaid with Rib Rolls (page 118), Oblique Curls with Rib Rolls (page 109), Opening Doors with Flexion and Extension (page 116).

Your *Immune* Health

In *Immunity: The Science of Staying Well*, Dr Jenna Macciochi describes the immune system as 'a mighty system' which 'protects our health by resisting uninvited infections, maintaining order and balance in our bodies and healing wounds. It is our foundation to wellbeing'. Your immune system attacks any 'invader' it sees as 'not belonging to you', viewing it as potentially dangerous. It is a highly complicated, finely-tuned and balanced system. When it does fail, either under- or overreacting to danger, you may succumb to a wide range of illnesses, from the common cold to cancer, autoimmune diseases, allergies, even mental health problems.

Joseph Pilates was no stranger to ill health. As a child, he suffered from rheumatic fever, rickets and asthma; all serious conditions back in the 1880s. His parents were warned he may not survive childhood. He proved them wrong: not only did he survive, but he became a fitness guru and always believed his method helped fight disease. Pilates was living in London at the outbreak of the First World War, and as he was German by birth, was interned in a prisoner of war camp. According to John Steele in *The Caged Lion*, Joe spent a lot of time in solitary confinement. When out of his cell, he took it upon himself to teach a daily exercise class. Pilates always claimed that his exercises prevented any of the prisoners dying from the Spanish flu epidemic, which claimed the lives of millions.

Current clients feel equally passionate about the health benefits of Pilates. In a recent survey, the main reason people took up Pilates was to manage a specific medical condition, but the main reason given for continuing was 'improved health and wellbeing'.[16]

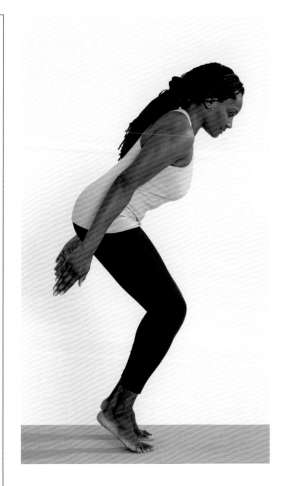

While we are on the topic of immune health, let us summarise the main foods that help. Try to ensure you are getting enough vitamins C and D, omega-3s and fibre. Eat as wide a range of foods as possible, including naturally colourful ingredients, in particular dark leafy vegetables and sulphur-rich alliums, like onions and garlic, plus cruciferous vegetables, such as cabbage, broccoli and cauliflower. Keeping your gut microbiome healthy is equally important (page 27).

LET THE LYMPH FLOW

According to Dr Macciochi, 'If you don't own your lymph, you don't own your health'. She also cites 'under-moving' as a contributory factor in poor immune health. One of the benefits of regular Pilates is the impact it has on the lymphatic system. Why is this important? We have seen how the lumphatic system plays a surveillance role in the body. If it detects a problem, it will transport vital white blood cells to the relevant site to tackle it. This, often overlooked, system consists of a huge network of nodes and vessels distributed throughout the body. With the exception of your nails, hair and cartilage, you are literally swimming in lymph fluid. This fluid, called chyle, transports many of your immune cells, proteins and hormones. It also acts as the body's waste disposal system.

During normal metabolic processes, cells produce waste products that need to be removed so that cells stay healthy and nutrients can reach them. The lymph 'collects' these toxins, which are then are filtered out by lymph nodes situated around the body. This lymph is then carried by vessels back to the thoracic ducts (just by the collarbones), where the cleaned lymph is returned to the bloodstream. Vital work, but even though it has millions of vessels, the lymphatic system has no strong pump, like the heart, to keep lymph moving. Instead, lymph is moved by breathing, walking, intestinal activity and muscle action. Lack of physical activity, sitting still for long periods, especially sitting slumped and breathing poorly, may result in lymph flow becoming sluggish. You want the lymph to flow freely. A lot of lymph tissue is situated in the centre of your body and every breath creates a vacuum effect, which helps lymph flow. So, when you practise deep breathing and focus on controlling your breathing during exercise, you are not only making your breathing more efficient, but also improving the function of your lymphatic system.

The other way to work on your lymphatic system is to get your joints moving. The rhythmic movements of Pilates are great at stimulating blood and lymph flow. As your muscles contract and release, lymph vessels are squeezed and lymph is pushed along and filtered through lymph nodes on its way back to the veins and heart. All physical activity is good for your lymphatic system, but Pilates is exceptionally good because it works the whole body, reaching parts you may not even realise you have!

While you have 600–1,000 lymph nodes situated all over your body, you have certain areas where they are found in clusters: the neck; under your arms; in your chest; abdomen and groin. It should come as no surprise that we will be targeting these areas. All exercises for a healthy immune system have been specifically chosen to get lymph flowing. Many of these exercises are new to Pilates, while others have been tweaked to make them more effective at encouraging lymph flow.

OVERTRAINING & THE IMMUNE SYSTEM

While we want you to move more, athletes, especially, need to take care not to overtrain. Overtraining is thought to have a negative impact on the immune system.[17] There are enormous health benefits associated with regular exercise but if you overdo it, you risk increased levels of norepinephrine and cortisol, the stress hormones, suppressing your immune system. Endurance athletes, including marathon runners and triathletes, are, for example, particularly prone to upper respiratory tract infections.

Always take note of how you feel after exercise, especially longer bouts (clearly not a problem with this programme!). Give your body a chance to recover. And remember, rest is just as important as activity.

A Balanced Life

Moving more, controlled breathing practices and good vagal tone are all vital for better health but they are not enough. They need to be accompanied by other lifestyle choices: good nutrition, weight management, cardiovascular activities for heart health (page 200), getting enough sunlight and darkness and a restful night's sleep. Joseph Pilates wrote of the importance of diet and sleep. We often forget just how essential sleep is. It is when your body repairs and recovers. It allows your blood pressure to regulate itself and thus impacts heart health.[18] It is linked to brain functions, including concentration and cognition. It helps to reduce inflammation. One study[19] showed that sleep patterns affect the hormones that control appetite. Not surprisingly, it also affects mental health.[20]

One of the secrets of a good night's sleep is to tune yourself into your natural circadian rhythm. Your circadian rhythm affects brainwave activity, hormone production, cell regeneration and many other biological processes. This internal clock affects your sleepiness, wakefulness and hunger. Production of hormones such as melatonin and cortisol can increase or decrease as part of your circadian rhythm. Your environment, body temperature, how long you work, your physical activity, all affect your circadian rhythm. As you age, your circadian rhythm changes. Babies develop their rhythm after a few months. Anyone who has tried to wake a sleeping teenager knows that they have their own body clock! Our circadian rhythms settle into a more consistent pattern as adults. Not surprisingly, it can be upset by shift work. Then as you get older, your body clock changes again and you get tired earlier and wake earlier.

'Epidemiological studies are consistently revealing more and more connection between modern lifestyles and our internal biological clock, and, when these two clash, it can lead to development of diseases such as obesity and breast cancer.'

STEVE KAY, PROFESSOR OF NEUROLOGY, BIOMEDICAL ENGINEERING AND BIOLOGICAL SCIENCES, UNIVERSITY OF SOUTHERN CALIFORNIA.

A word about napping. A study at Shanghai Jiao Tong University revealed that afternoon naps of just 5 minutes helped memory and brain agility (cognitive function). If you need a longer nap, set an alarm for 40 minutes; after this time your body will get deeper into sleep meaning if you wake you may still feel groggy, or set the alarm for 2 hours to enable your body to enter a deep sleep cycle. If you're having trouble sleeping, try skipping the afternoon nap.

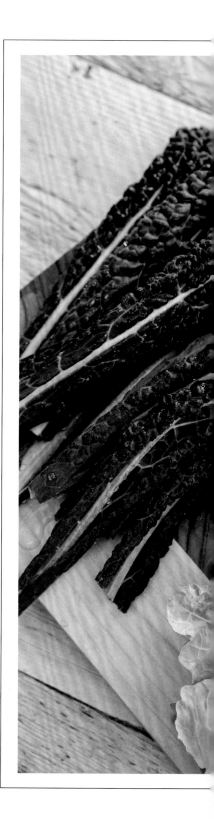

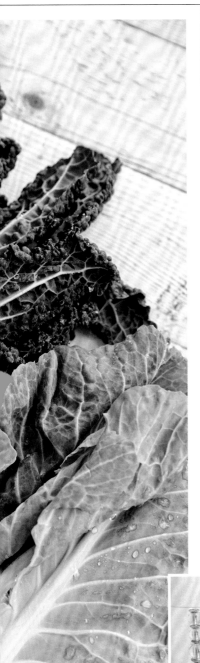

A Healthy Balanced Diet

If you have read *Shape Up with Pilates*, you will know about my personal adage regarding nutrition: 'Eat first what you should, and then what you would'. This has stood me in good stead all my adult life. Finding the right balance in your diet is crucial. I know I should eat plenty of wholegrains, nuts, seeds, seasonal and local fresh fruit and vegetables, especially leafy green ones, pulses, lean proteins, in particular, plenty of fresh, responsibly sourced fish and some dairy. Then I leave what I would eat (and drink) – dark chocolate, a glass of red wine and, yes, the occasional medicinal gin – until the evenings as a reward for eating healthily all day!

Whenever possible, I try to eat food that is unprocessed and contains no unnecessary additives. Fortunately, I love cooking, or rather I love feeding people, so I usually prepare meals from scratch. I have never cut out a complete food group as I'm lucky not to have intolerances or allergies.

Variety is key. In 1985, the Japanese government, in an attempt to counter the negative influence of the increasingly popular western diet, advised its population to 'Consume 30 different food items each day'. If you can manage this, it should help ensure you get all the nutrients your body needs. I also try to eat a rainbow of colourful fruits and veg.

There is increasing evidence of the importance of the gut microbiome to your overall health. The microbiome is the collective name for the bacteria, viruses and fungi that live inside us. These bacteria play a key role in the health of your immune system, brain and even influence your weight. Up to 1,000 species of bacteria reside in the human gut microbiome; the majority are beneficial, but there are some that can cause disease. It is clear we need to encourage the 'good' guys and deter the 'bad' ones. An imbalance is sometimes referred to as gut dysbiosis and may contribute to weight gain, which is why taking probiotics daily is so important for both mental and physical health.[21]

But now, it's time to get you moving with the Pilates Express® programme.

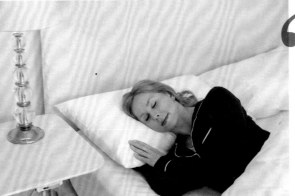

> "
> *'Suicide by lifestyle takes ages.'*
>
> ———
>
> BILL BRYSON,
> *THE BODY:
> A GUIDE FOR
> OCCUPANTS*

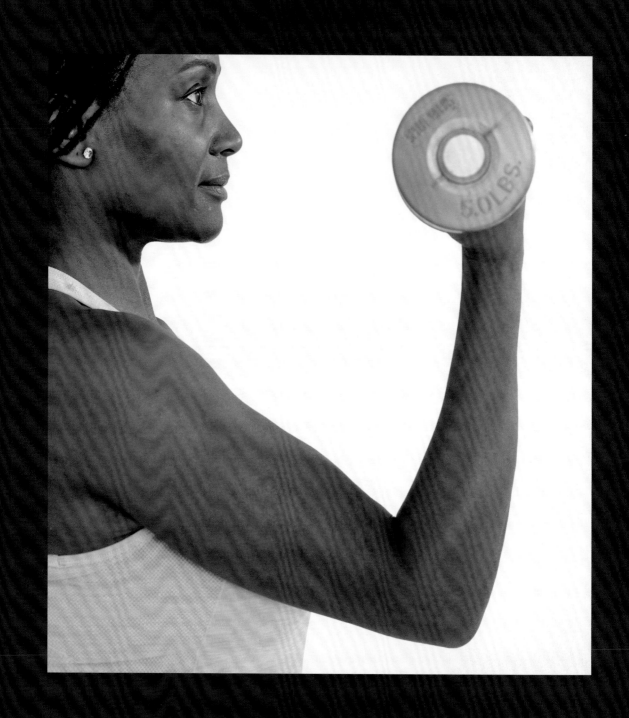

The *Pilates Express®* Programme

CHAPTER ONE

Before You *Begin*

Everything you need to know for good Pilates practice is contained within the next two chapters.

Before you start to exercise, read through Tips for Good Practice and then go straight to The New Fundamentals (page 33). This is a deal breaker, even if you have done Pilates before. We are constantly updating our teaching of The Fundamentals, so recommend revisiting them regularly. This is the equivalent of reading a recipe through, checking you have the right pots, pans and ingredients before you start cooking! Many of the combination exercises in the programme use exercises from The New Fundamentals, so you will need to know them.

Once the New Fundamentals are mastered, you can then start on the Exercises for Respiratory Health, Exercises for a Healthy Immune System and finally the Strength and Flexibility Exercises. When you are ready to start the workouts, you will find that they use exercises from each of these chapters as well as The New Fundamentals.

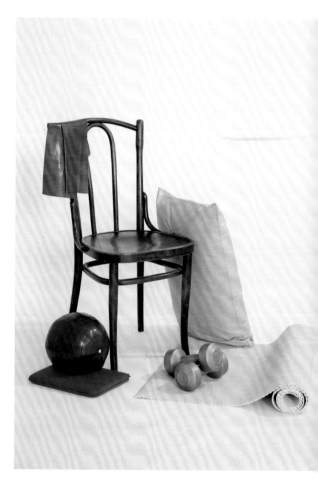

HERE IS A LIST OF THE EQUIPMENT YOU ARE GOING TO NEED:

- Padded non-slip mat
- Folded towel or small flat pillow
- Bed pillow
- Stretch band of medium strength, preferably a long one or a long stretchy scarf
- Sturdy chair
- Clear stretch of wall space
- Hand weights. How heavy they are depends on several factors: primarily your technique, which must never be compromised. Then it depends on what you want to achieve and what the goals of the exercise are. Traditionally, we do not use heavy weights in Pilates as they restrict flowing movement and risk bulking muscles. We would prefer not to set you a particular weight limit, it is better that you gradually build up strength, without losing control.

If you do not have weights, you can use cans or bottles of water.

TIPS FOR GOOD PILATES PRACTICE

Good practice = maximum results.

- If exercising indoors, always prepare the space by making it warm, comfortable and free from distractions. Make sure that you have enough room to move your arms and legs. If you like, you can play some background music, but it should be quiet and not distracting.

- Wear clothing that allows freedom of movement but that will also allow you to check your alignment. Barefoot is best, but you can also wear non-slip socks. If outside or at work, you may wear shoes but preferably ones with a flexible sole so that you can roll through your feet correctly.

- See page 185 for Tips on Exercising Outdoors.

- Remember your **ABC**s – **A**lignment, **B**reathing and **C**entring – at all times.

- Read through each exercise carefully. We have given you the main focus of the exercise in the **Challenges and Benefits**; this may include the area of the body that it targets, a movement skill or both!

- Always take time to find the correct Starting Alignment as this will impact the precision of your movements. You will find the different Starting Positions, such as Relaxation Position, Four-point Kneeling etc. in the Alignment section on pages 34-35. Note that if your Starting Position is not right, your movement path will not be right.

- Your Starting Position will also be your Finishing Position. Returning to the Starting Position with precision and control after each repetition or at the end of the exercise sequence is as important as the exercise itself.

- For some exercises, you have a choice of Starting Position. We have utilised this to help keep your workouts varied. Some of these Starting Positions will increase the challenge and difficulty of the exercise considerably.

- Make sure that you fully understand all the movements described in the Action Points. If you look at the photographs that accompany them, you will see that they provide the sequence of movements. They will also give you a visual image of what you are trying to achieve.

- In an ideal world, you would have a well-qualified teacher helping you to find perfect alignment and checking you are moving correctly. However, when you are working alone, you have to check yourself. The Watchpoints give you extra tips on how to perfect your technique and avoid common pitfalls. You might find it helpful to check your alignment in a mirror.

- Do read the section on page 36 about your **Centreline**. This is your axis. Awareness of it can help you find the right alignment before you start, help you centre yourself and ensure you maintain good alignment while you move. Control of axial movement is paramount.

- When trying the breathing exercises, allow yourself time to adjust and absorb the new patterns. *Note that some people can become anxious when trying to control their breathing. If this is the case, stop immediately.* You do not have to do breathing exercises at all. You can simply try the other exercises, focusing on the movements rather than the breathing.

- Try to start with a different leg, arm or side each time you practise. We all favour one side, so it is good to balance this out.

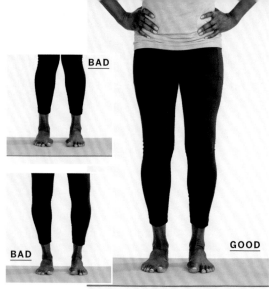

- The number of repetitions given is the ideal number for you to work towards. However, it is quality over quantity every time please. If your technique is suffering because muscles are fatiguing, stop and rest. You can always revisit the exercise later. Time will also be a factor here. If you are keeping strictly to the 10 minutes rule, you may have to limit the number of repetitions. As you become more familiar with the exercises, it will get easier to fit them all in.

- Talking of balancing out, if you are doing a one-legged or one-armed exercise it's also a good idea to do one repetition on two legs or two arms to finish.

- Leg Alignment – When you bend your knees, for example in a Squat or Lunge, we will give you the direction to bend them over your second toes. This is to help you achieve correct hip, knee and ankle alignment. We do not want you to roll your knees and ankles in or out.

- Similarly, when you lift your heels to come up onto your toes, for example in Walking on the Spot, page 132, direct the front of your ankles forwards over your second toes and roll through your feet, lifting your heels to bring your weight onto the balls of your feet. Your toes remain grounded, without gripping the floor, keeping them active.

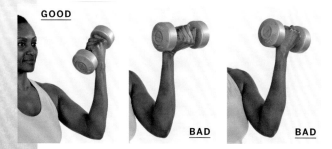

- When using hand-held weights or a band, keep good wrist alignment as shown below.

- If you wish to use weights, it is important to first warm up your large joints (we have planned for this in the workouts). Practise without weights first, then gradually increase the weight over time, but not at the expense of good technique! Men can usually lift heavier weights without losing technique. Use your judgement.

- One of the key features of this programme is time saving, so you will see we use the direction '**simultaneously**' frequently in the Action Points. This is usually when we want you to combine movements. Initially, practise the movements separately for a few repetitions and then combine them, so that you can retain the quality of each movement.

- Do not be tempted to speed up the exercises. It is better, and more challenging, to slow them down. Try a Curl Up quickly and then slowly and you will see what we mean.

- The devil is in the detail. With Pilates, you have to sweat the small stuff, it's important.

- See page 185 for advice on working out outdoors.

PLEASE DO NOT EXERCISE IF:

- You are feeling unwell.
- You have just eaten a heavy meal.
- You have been drinking alcohol.
- You are in pain from injury. Always consult your practitioner first, as rest may be needed before exercise.
- You have been taking strong painkillers, as it will mask any warning signs.
- You are undergoing medical treatment or are taking medication. Again, you will need to consult your practitioner first.

Remember, it is always wise to consult your doctor before taking up a new exercise regime. If you have a medical condition, this is essential.

The New Fundamentals

The following pages are, without question, the most important pages in the book. Skip them at your peril!

These fundamentals will ensure, not only that you are working correctly, but also that you get the maximum benefit from the exercises. Even if you are a Pilates veteran, you should still revisit these exercises on a regular basis. Our method is constantly evolving, taking on board new scientific research, so it is good to stay updated.

Do not think of the ABCs of Alignment, Breathing and Centring as being just for the start of a session. They need to be incorporated into every move you make. But first, let's put them in context. The ABCs are taken from Body Control Pilates' Eight Principles, which underpin our whole approach.

1. **CONCENTRATION**
2. **RELAXATION**
3. **ALIGNMENT**
4. **BREATHING**
5. **CENTRING**
6. **CO-ORDINATION**
7. **FLOWING MOVEMENTS**
8. **STAMINA**

In a nutshell, we want you to be: fully focused on what you are doing, mindful of every movement; free from unnecessary tension; in the best possible position before you start an exercise, while you move and also in the best postural alignment as you go about your daily activities; breathing as efficiently as you can; stable and centred in your movements (and in your life!); co-ordinated and in control of your movements; moving freely with ease and flow; full of energy, vim and vigour with sufficient stamina to enjoy life!

All this is possible with regular Pilates practice. But the areas that we will be focusing on in this chapter are what we call The Fundamentals: how to find good postural Alignment in a variety of positions, how to Breathe efficiently during the exercises and how to stay Centred while you move.

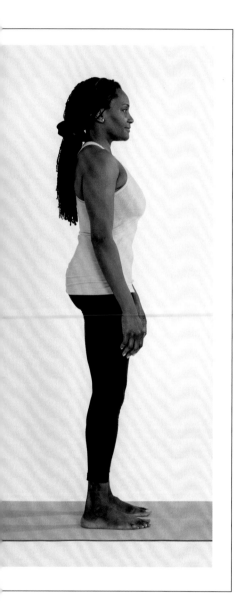

Alignment

Why is good posture important? Joseph Pilates saw poor posture as a common problem:

'Note daily the thousands of persons with round, stooped shoulders and protruding abdomens.'

——————————— RETURN TO LIFE

He believed good postural alignment to be, not just better for your movement, but also important for your health:

Apart from the above, poor alignment places a strain on your joints, resulting in uneven wear and tear. It can cause muscles to be out of balance. And – this might just be the deciding factor for you – your posture also has a dramatic impact on how you look.

If you have ever caught sight of yourself slouching in a mirror, you will know it is not a pretty sight. Strange how we usually pull ourselves up tall when we check our reflection! But then what happens when we walk away from the mirror? Do we continue to stand up straight? Most of us, in the absence of a visual reminder like a mirror, friendly Pilates teacher or Mary Poppins, tend to revert to slouching.

Try both slouching and then standing tall in front of a mirror and see the difference.

'... the slouch position... upsets the equilibrium of the body resulting in disarrangement of the various organs affected including the bones and muscles of the body as well as the nerves and blood vessels, not overlooking the glands.'

——————————— YOUR HEALTH

SLOUCHED:

01/ Your stomach sticks out

02/ Your waist disappears as your ribs sink towards your hips

03/ You appear shorter

Good posture will be discussed at length later (page 50) but for now, lengthen up through the crown of your head, open your shoulders, allow your arms to relax down by your sides. For a moment, gently draw your lower abdominals back toward your spine. Breathe.

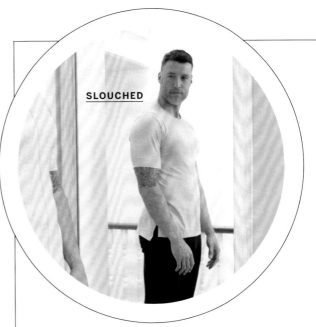

SLOUCHED

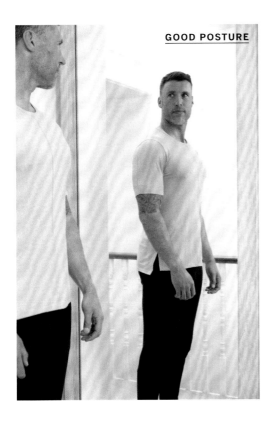

GOOD POSTURE

GOOD POSTURE:
OBSERVE THE CHANGES:

01/ You look instantly taller

02/ Your waist has reappeared

03/ Your stomach looks flatter

The problem is that, for most of us, standing tall is very tiring. It requires inner strength from your deep postural muscles to keep you upright. Your deep 'core' muscles are basically anti-gravity muscles. When they are weak, it is very difficult to have good posture all day. Pilates can give you this inner postural strength, the ability to stand tall easily, without effort, day in, day out. This is what has drawn performers to Pilates for years. Imagine the physical strain of being on stage or in front of the camera all day.

But there is more to good posture than good alignment of the bones and efficient core muscles. You need to 'feel' good posture, understand it and experience it.

This chapter will help you position yourself in good alignment for your Starting Positions. Remember too that you need to stay in control of your alignment whilst you move through the exercises.

Your Centreline

Before we describe the Starting Positions, a word about your Centreline. This is the vertical axis of your body. We have already noted the mental health benefits that accompany 'control of axial body movement and posture' (page 21). Moving through, along and around your Centreline, is essential to your control of good alignment. And remember, we are aiming for axial length at all times. But first you need to identify your Centreline.

You can see from the image opposite that we have dropped a plumbline down from the nose, through the notch at the base of your neck, through your breastbone, navel, centre of your pubic bone to fall precisely at a mid-point between your feet.

Please remember, to quote my favourite physiotherapist 'We are trees not lampposts!' Very few of us are this symmetrical. Believe us when we say it took a while to get our model into such a symmetrical position. If you have a scoliosis, a curvature of the spine, it is just as valuable to visualise your Centreline and work around it.

While it may be difficult for us to achieve this degree of symmetry in the body, if we can work towards it, it will help to balance muscles and align joints in their neutral, mid-position, zones. Balanced muscles are more likely to be the right length and strength to work together to move us. Well-aligned joints are better able to withstand the stresses and strains of everyday living.

Many of the exercises involve you moving around this Centreline, creating axial length. Keep it in mind whenever you twist, when rolling through it as you curl or uncurl, and then, return to it when you have completed your movements. This will then help you work correctly, as well as helping your stress levels. Initially, you will need to keep checking your alignment. Ultimately, you should be able to sense it.

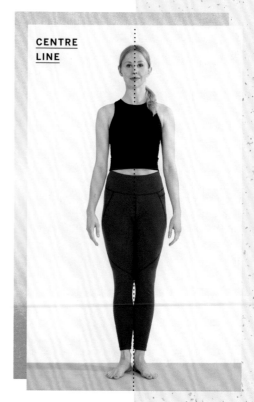

CENTRE LINE

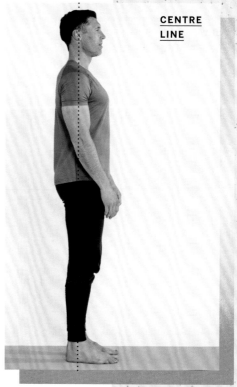

CENTRE LINE

Starting (*and* Finishing) Positions

RELAXATION POSITION

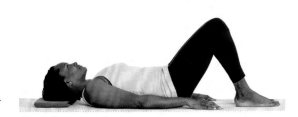

Here we will explain the different Starting Positions in the programme. Remember, they are also the Finishing Positions too. And remember, you should stay in control of your alignment throughout the exercise. The easiest place to learn good alignment is in The Relaxation Position, because the ground will give you feedback, helping you find the right position.

Relaxation Position

Relaxation Position is both an exercise and the Starting and Finishing Position for many of the lying exercises. It is one of the most important positions to get right. As an exercise, Relaxation Position can be used to release tension, improve body awareness for good postural alignment, breathing and stability. As a Starting Position, use it to check your ABCs.

Starting Position

Lie on your back on the mat with your knees bent, feet hip-width apart and parallel. Aim your heels towards the centre of each buttock and your feet should be about hip-width apart. If you need to, place a small, folded towel or firm, flat pillow underneath your head. The idea is for your neck to be lengthened but to maintain its natural curve. Your head should be neither tipped forward nor back. Sometimes a pillow is not necessary, or you may need a couple.

If you are going to 'remain' in Relaxation Position, place your hands on the lower abdomen to allow the shoulders to widen and open. You could pop a pillow under each elbow to help with tension release. If you are using Relaxation Position as a Starting Position, have your arms relaxed by your sides, palms facing the floor.

WATCHPOINTS

- Allow your entire spine to widen and lengthen as it relaxes and feels supported by the mat.

- Focus on three areas of body weight: your ribcage, pelvis and head.

- Be aware of your body parts touching the mat and encourage them to feel heavy and supported. You will feel less contact with the mat in your lower spine.

- Allow your thighs to sink down towards your hips, your lower legs towards the ankles and allow your feet to be grounded.

- Focus on the width across your chest and feel released in the breastbone.

- Feel lengthened in your neck and soften your jaw and forehead.

- Allow time for your body to settle and spine to release.

When coming out of this position, please roll onto your side and rest a moment before coming up.

Compass

This exercise helps you develop an awareness of neutral alignment around the pelvis and lower spine. It is also a great way to mobilise and release the lower back.

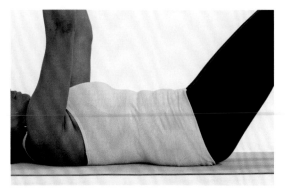

Relaxation Position (note: photo presents arms lifted to show spinal alignment), arms lengthened along your sides on the mat. Imagine there is a compass on your lower abdomen; your navel represents north, your pubic bone south and the prominent bones of your pelvis are west and east.

ACTION

01/ Breathe in to prepare.

02/ Breathe out as you gently tilt your pelvis to the north (the pubic bone moves forwards and up). Feel your lower spine release into the mat as your pelvis tilts back.

03/ Breathe in as you tilt your pelvis back through the mid-position, without stopping, until the pelvis tilts gently forwards to the south (the pubic bone moves backwards and down). Your lower back will arch slightly.

Repeat this north/south tilt x 5.

04/ Return to the Starting Position and find your neutral position, which is the mid-position – neither north nor south but in between.

05/ Breathe out as you roll your pelvis to one side – west. Feel the opposite side of the pelvis lift slightly as the pelvis rotates. Try to roll directly to the side without shortening one side of your waist (that is, without hip hiking).

06/ Breathe in as you roll your pelvis through the mid-position, without stopping, to the other side – east. Feel the opposite side of your pelvis lift slightly as your pelvis rotates.

07/ Return to the mid-position. Your pelvis is level. This is your neutral position.

When coming out of this position, please roll onto your side and rest a moment before coming up.

WATCHPOINTS

• Tilting should be easy and comfortable.

• The final position of neutral should feel natural, not held or fixed.

• The back of the pelvis should feel heavy and grounded into the mat.

• Your waist is equally lengthened on both sides.

• Ensure that there is equal weight on both sides of the pelvis.

• Allow your hip joints to be free and released.

• Once you have found neutral pelvis, do not forget about the rest of the body. Run through all of the Watchpoints for Relaxation Position (page 37).

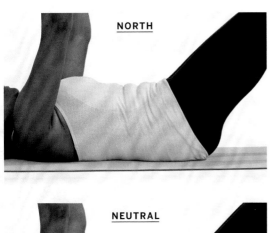

NORTH

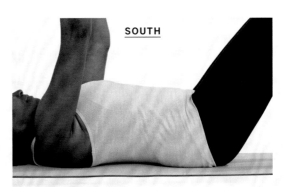

SOUTH

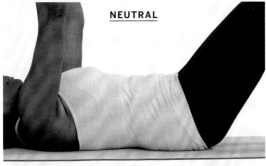

NEUTRAL

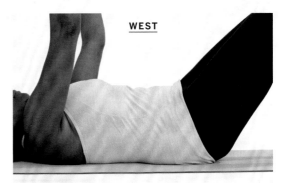

WEST

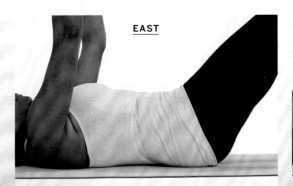

EAST

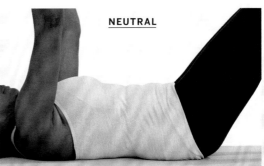

NEUTRAL

QUICK NEUTRAL CHECK

Place your hands on your lower abdomen, forming a triangle. Your fingertips touch your pubic bone and the base of your thumbs rest approximately on your prominent pelvic bones. When you are in neutral, your hands are parallel to the floor (tummy permitting) and both sides of your waist are equal in length. Now you can focus more specifically on the correct alignment of the head and neck relative to the rest of your spine.

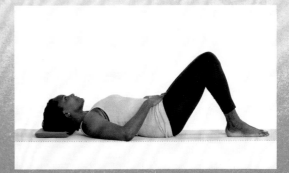

Chin Tucks *and* Neck Rolls

This is another Compass-style exercise but for the head and neck. You will roll the head through the different positions, coming to rest in a mid, neutral position. This exercise develops an awareness of neutral alignment around the head and neck and is an effective way to release tension there. Perfect for the warm-up of your workouts.

STARTING POSITION

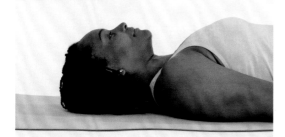

Relaxation Position (page 37). You can also do Neck Rolls and Chin Tucks in upright positions, but you will not have the support or feedback from the floor so you will need to be extra vigilant about the positioning of your head on top of your lengthened spine.

ACTION

01/ Breathe in to prepare.

02/ Breathe out as you lengthen the back of the neck and nod your head forwards, drawing the chin down. Keep your head in contact with the mat.

03/ Breathe in as you tip your head back gently, passing through the mid-position without stopping, to slightly extend your neck. Keep the back of your head in contact with the mat as the chin glides up; this is a small and subtle movement.

04/ Repeat the above x 5 and then find the mid-position where your head is neither tipped back or forwards and your neck is neither flexed nor extended. This is neutral, with your face and your focus both directed towards the ceiling.

05/ Breathe out as you keep your neck released and roll your head to one side. Again, make sure that you keep your head in contact with the mat.

06/ Breathe in as you roll your head back to the centre.

Repeat to the other side and repeat the Neck Roll up to x 5 before returning your head to the centre with even length on both sides of your neck.

WATCHPOINTS

• Keep your neck long throughout.

• The movements are small and should feel comfortable.

• As you draw your chin down, ensure that the back of your head slides along the mat as opposed to simply pressing the back of the neck into the mat.

• Try not to disturb the natural, neutral curves of your upper and lower back.

• Alternate which side you roll to each time you include the exercise in a workout.

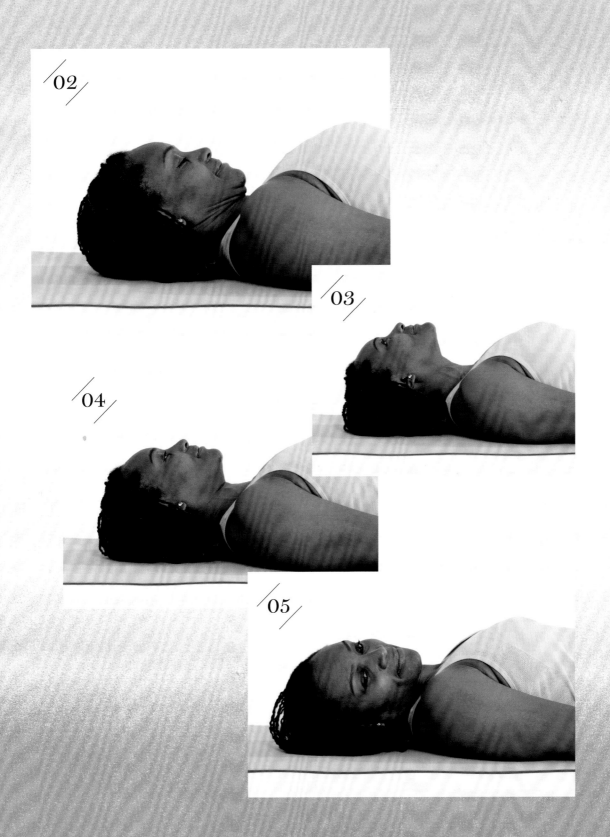

Seated Starting Postitions

You will find a variety of Seated Starting Positions in the book. The arm and leg positions vary.

Seated on a Mat —— *or Long Frog*

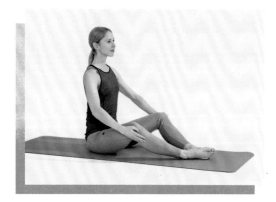

Sit upright on the mat. You may be more comfortable sitting on a rolled-up towel or cushion as this helps you into a neutral spine position. Bend your knees, turn your legs out from the hips and connect the soles of your feet. Your feet should be quite a distance from the body to allow a feeling of space in the hip joints. Place your hands on your shins; your arms are lengthened but elbows are slightly bent. Have your head balanced centrally over your ribcage, ribcage over your pelvis.

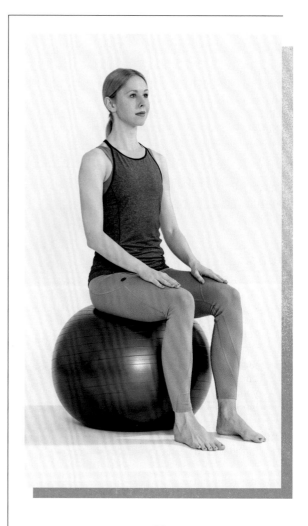

Sitting on a Ball

If you are lucky enough to be able to sit on a physio/Swiss ball at your desk, your core muscles will be working naturally to keep you upright. They can tire so do take short breaks from the ball and be aware of sitting tall – do not slouch. You may need your feet wider apart to help you balance. You should still be able to do most of the Seated Workouts on page 186 but much will depend on your stability and balance. Be safe and don't fall off!

Seated on a Chair

We are going to take a close look at alignment when you are sitting in a chair. For your Midday Workouts (pages 186–93), you may be at work and unable to leave your desk. We should just reiterate that sitting for long periods is not good for your health so, unless it is unavoidable, always opt for alternative positions.

The type of chair makes a difference. It should be sturdy and, if possible, without arms so you can include exercises where you swing your arms.

ACTION

01/ Sit tall on your chair, feet grounded on the floor, hip-width apart and parallel. Your knees should be bent at about 90 degrees, the lower part of your legs perpendicular and heels lined up with the back of the knees. You may need to place your feet on a low platform (or a couple of large books) to achieve this.

02/ Check that your weight is evenly balanced in the centre of both sitting bones.

03/ We are aiming for an elongated 'S' shape for the spine, not a collapsed 'C' shape. Check that you have a gentle hollow in the lower back (lumbar lordosis). Avoid rolling back onto your coccyx, which would take you into a slouched 'C' shape. Similarly, avoid rolling too far forwards onto your pubic bone, which causes the lower back to overarch. Lengthen up through the whole spine so that the subtle natural curves are kept.

04/ Your ribcage should be directly above the pelvis, neither swaying backwards nor slumping forwards.

05/ Place your fingertips on your sternum and gently lift through this area to ensure good posture.

06/ Feel your shoulder blades wide in the upper back and collarbones open in the front of the chest.

07/ Lengthen your neck and allow your head to balance freely on top of the spine.

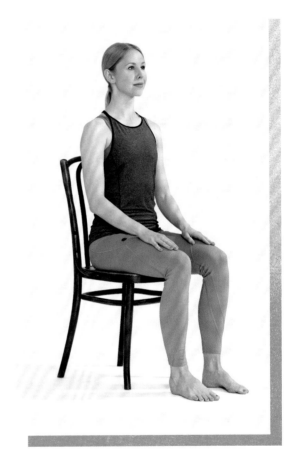

It is not easy to maintain this elongated 'S' shape while seated, but regular Pilates practice will help. In the meantime, if it is more comfortable and your chair has a back, you can place a small support in the lumbar curve. A rolled-up towel or even a small ball inflated to about 25 per cent can work well. Remove this support when doing exercises like Seated Cat.

EXERCISE

Four-point Kneeling

You cannot just rest in this position – you need to be active!

STARTING POSITION

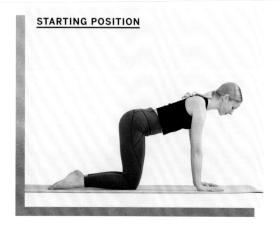

Kneel on all fours on the mat. Position your hands directly underneath your shoulders and knees directly beneath your hips.

WATCHPOINTS

• As with Compass (page 38), the tilting of your pelvis is small. The rest of your spine will react slightly, but do not over-exaggerate this.

• Fully lengthen your arms but avoid locking your elbows.

• Keep your collarbones wide, your neck free of tension.

ACTION

Finding neutral pelvis and spine:

01/ Breathe in and lengthen your spine.

02/ Breathe out as you tilt your pelvis backwards (north – your tailbone curls under) allowing your lower back to slightly round (flex).

03/ Breathe in and lengthen the spine and tilt your pelvis forwards (south – your tailbone sticks out) allowing your lower back to slightly arch (extend).

Repeat x 3, then find the mid-position where your pelvis is neutral. This position is lengthened and level, neither tucked nor arched.

Allow for the natural curvature of the lumbar spine, finding good shoulder alignment to free the neck from tension:

04/ Breathe in and keeping your elbows straight, gently draw your shoulder blades together (retracting them). Your upper spine will lower slightly toward the mat.

05/ Breathe out as you allow your shoulder blades to glide wider on your ribcage (protracting them). Your upper spine will round slightly.

Repeat x 3, then find the mid-position of the shoulder blades between these two extremes. Allow for the natural curvature of your upper spine and neck. Lengthen your whole spine from your crown to tailbone.

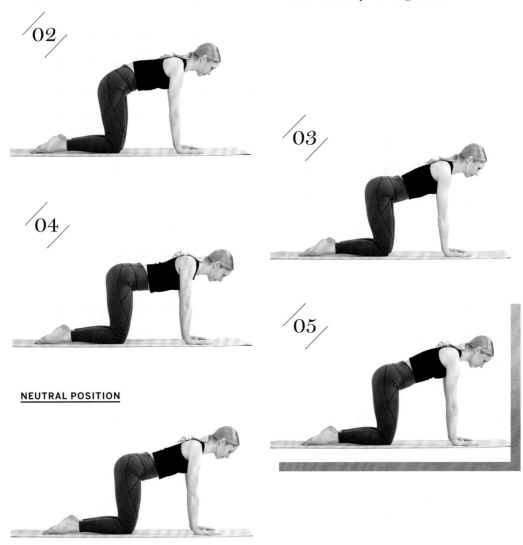

02

03

04

NEUTRAL POSITION

05

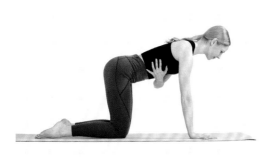

Three-point Kneeling

To add challenge, try Three-point Kneeling, which means taking one arm away, reducing your support.

Normally for this position, you wrap the non-supporting arm around your ribs.

Note that in this position you will need to work extra hard to keep your shoulders wide and open and your pelvis square and neutral. And when you move your spine, the challenge will be to keep to the Centreline!

EXERCISE

High Kneeling

Not everyone finds this position comfortable. If it does not suit you, try Standing (page 50) instead.

High kneel on a padded mat (to protect your knees) but not so padded you feel unstable. Have your knees hip-width apart and, if you wish, place a small cushion between the thighs (the cushion should be about hip-width in thickness). Ensure that your weight falls not just through the knees but through the length of both shins evenly.

ACTION

01/ Lengthen up through your spine.

02/ Lengthen your waist equally on both sides.

03/ Position your ribcage directly above your neutral pelvis, neither swaying backwards, nor slumping forwards.

04/ Feel your shoulder blades wide in the upper back and collarbones open in the front of the chest.

05/ Place your fingertips on your sternum and gently lift up through this area. Relax your hands but stay 'lifted'.

06/ Allow your arms to hang freely in the shoulder sockets. Feel space underneath the armpits and a sense of length and weight through the hands.

07/ Release your neck and allow your head to balance freely on top of the spine. Sense the crown of the head lengthening up to the ceiling.

08/ Relax your jaw and focus directly forwards.

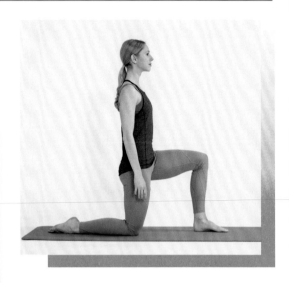

High-kneeling Lunge Position

If you are not happy in this position, try High Kneeling or Split Stance Standing (page 52).

To get into the High-kneeling Lunge, start by following the directions above (minus the cushion), then bring one leg in front of you in line with your hip. Have your knee bent directly over your ankle at 90 degrees.

WATCHPOINTS

• Take care not to press forwards into your hips, keep your pelvis, ribcage and head stacked vertically over each other.

• It is worth checking your knee and ankle alignment during the exercises as it is easy to lose the 90-degree angle.

• Your hip bones are level.

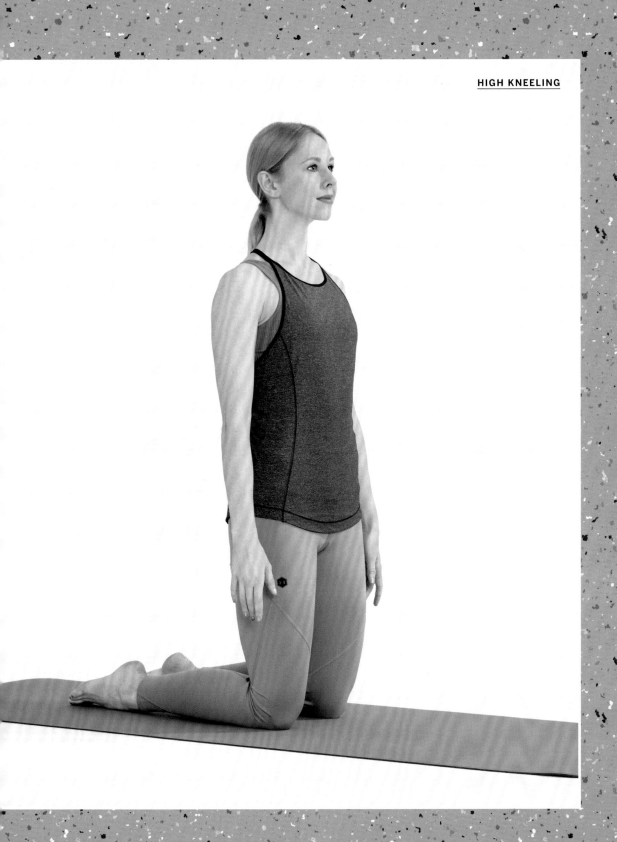

EXERCISE

Prone Starting Positions

Diamond Press

Lie on your front in a straight line. Create a diamond shape with the arms. Place the fingertips together, palms down on the mat and open your elbows. Rest your forehead on the backs of your hands. If it is more comfortable, widen your hands to allow your shoulders to broaden and relax (you may need a folded towel under your forehead if you do this). Your legs are hip-width apart and parallel.

You will find a variety of Prone Starting Positions in the book – Dart (page 119), Full Star (page 146) and Cobra Prep (page 91) all have different arm and leg positions.

DART STARTING POSITION

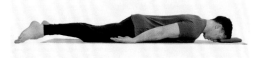

DIAMOND PRESS STARTING POSITION

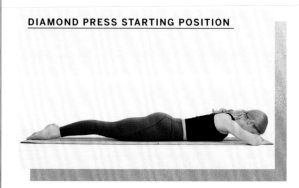

COBRA STARTING POSITION

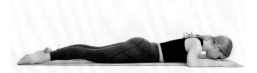

Always check that you are lying in a straight line – you can run tape down the centre of your mat to help.

WATCHPOINTS

- Avoid flattening or arching your lower spine; it should feel lengthened. If there is any discomfort there, you may place a very small, flat cushion or folded towel under your abdomen to support your spine.

- Think of connecting the front of your lower ribcage and the top of your pelvis. Focus on the heaviness of your ribs releasing into the mat.

- Allow your chest to be open and collarbones to widen.

- Keep your neck long and ensure that your chin is neither tucked in nor lifted up.

- Place a pillow under your shins if this helps (it is a good way to avoid cramp).

EXERCISE

Side-lying Starting Positions

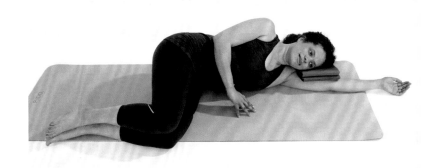

You will find a variety of Side-lying Starting Positions in the book. The head, arm and leg positions vary, and this sometimes changes the level of difficulty. The more your body is contact with the floor, the easier it will be as you will have more support.

Side-lying Chair

Lie on your side and bend both knees in front of you so that your hips and knees are bent to a right angle. Line up hip over hip, knee over knee, shoulder over shoulder. To help check you are straight, you can line your torso up with the back edge of your mat. You can place a pillow between your knees to bring your knees, ankles and feet in line with your hips as shown. This is particularly helpful if you have hip or back problems.

Your underneath arm is outstretched in line with your spine. You will need a flat cushion or folded towel between your head and arm to keep your head aligned. Men usually need more than one as their shoulders tend to be wider. Your top arm is bent, your hand resting gently in front of your torso to provide light support.

If you are doing an exercise such as Bow and Arrow on page 86, you can rest your head on a pillow so that the head and neck are aligned with the spine, and your arms are stretched out in front of you at shoulder height.

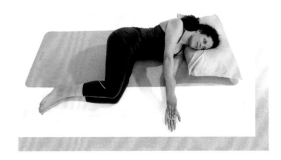

WATCHPOINTS

• Avoid your body rolling forwards or tipping back. Imagine that you are lying in between two panes of glass and stack yourself accordingly.

• Maintain the natural curves of the spine.

• Lengthen both sides of your waist equally; this is essential in Side Lying as it is very easy to allow the lower side of your spine to dip down towards the mat and your spine to collapse.

EXERCISE

Standing

Stand tall on the floor, feet hip-width apart in a natural stance, neither turned out nor in a rigid parallel position. Allow your arms to lengthen by your sides.

We want you standing tall 24/7 and to do this you need to practise and build endurance in your deep postural muscles. Stamina is one of our Eight Principles (page 33). Standing tall is a dynamic exercise rather than a 'position'.

We are aiming for 80 per cent of your body weight to be balanced over the arches of your feet. We have 18 Watchpoints to help you to stand well, so we are not taking any chances! It may help you to know that, when you stand tall, you are recruiting many of the deep postural muscles, the ones holding you up against gravity.

Visualise your Centreline (page 36).

WATCHPOINTS

• Lean forwards slightly from your ankle joint so that your weight shifts onto the balls of the feet, while the heels stay down.

• Lean backwards slightly from your ankle joint so that your weight shifts onto the heels; the toes should be lengthened and without tension.

• Place your weight over the arches in the centre of the feet and notice that there is a triangle of connection with the floor: a point at the base of the big toe, the little toe and the centre of the heel. The toes should be active.

• Lengthen your legs but allow your knees to soften.

• Tilt your pelvis forwards slightly (south so that your pubic bone moves back and your lower back slightly arches).

• Passing through neutral, slightly tilt your pelvis backwards (north so that your pubic bone moves forwards and your lower back slightly rounds).

• Return your pelvis to your neutral position, where the pubic bone is on same plane as your prominent pelvic bones, which are also level with each other.

• Lengthen your waist equally on both sides.

• Find your centre by gently recruiting your pelvic floor and deep abdominal muscles (page 36).

• Relax your ribcage and position it directly above the pelvis, neither swaying backwards, nor slumping forwards.

STARTING POSITION

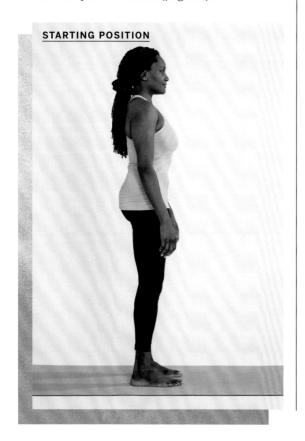

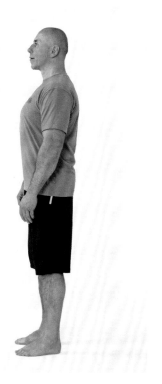

- Gently lift up through your breastbone.

- Feel your shoulder blades wide in the upper back and collarbones open in the front of the chest. Soften your breastbone.

- Allow your arms to hang freely in the shoulder sockets. Feel space underneath the armpits and a sense of length and weight through the hands.

- Release your neck and allow your head to balance freely on top of the spine. Sense the crown of the head lengthening up to the ceiling.

- Relax your jaw and focus directly forwards.

- While lengthening up, maintain a sense of what is happening in your lower body and be aware of the contact of your feet with the floor.

- Breathe naturally into the ribcage.

- This position should not feel forced or held but as if you are growing upwards dynamically.

EXERCISE

Pilates Stance

Pilates Stance is a standing position which is very useful to 'connect' to your deep core muscles and subtly engage deep gluteal and inner thigh muscles.

01/ Follow the directions above but have your legs slightly turned out from the hips, inner thighs connected, if possible (sometimes your leg shape does not allow this).

02/ Heels are also connected, if possible, and toes slightly apart, creating a small 'V' position with the feet.

03/ Your arms are relaxed by your sides.

04/ Connect the entire length of the inner thighs with a sense of drawing them together and up towards the pubic bone. If the inner thighs do not touch, do not force them.

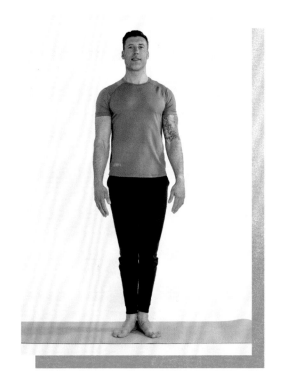

EXERCISE

Split Stance

For the first time in a book, we are going to include Split Stance in Alignment. While it is not a traditional Pilates Starting Position, we have been increasingly using Split Stance in our teaching. Why? It is very functional. We spend a lot of our day in a Split Stance, for example, when walking. It is very rare for us to stop in a daily activity and line our feet up hip-width apart in parallel!

We still need to practise exercises with our feet in line, as this promotes symmetry and balance in the body. However, it is also useful to occasionally challenge the body to cope with different positions, such as Split Stance.

Take note of the additional challenges Split Stance positions present. For example, whenever you are in a Split Stance, you will be challenging your ability to control rotation in your body. Awareness of axial length along your Centreline will help.

Where possible, the workouts start and finish in a parallel rather than a Split Stance position. This is to restore balance. Remember to do repetitions with the other foot forwards and try to vary which foot you place forwards first to avoid 'favouring' one foot over the other.

Split Stance Standing

Stand tall and take a step forwards with one foot. Do not step too far. You want to keep your trunk centred (remember your Centreline) and weight evenly distributed between your feet.

You can either turn out the back leg or keep it in parallel, whichever feels more natural to you. Now, let's apply Split Stance to other positions...

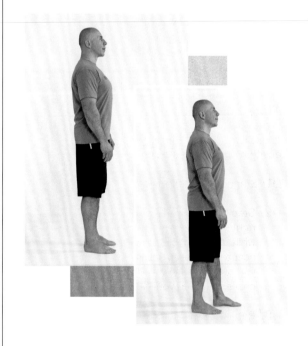

Split Stance Four-point Kneeling

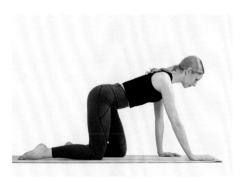

Follow the instructions for Four-point Kneeling (page 44) but stagger the position of either the hands or knees, or both. When staggering your hand position, ensure that your upper body is still well balanced between the hands and your shoulders remain wide and open. The same applies to staggering the knee position, only it is the pelvis that needs to stay centred. The pelvis will rotate slightly but try to stay true to your Centreline, weight even on both knees. If you are staggering hands and knees, stagger opposite ones, it is more natural.

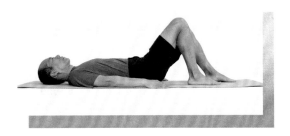

Split Stance in Relaxation Position

From Relaxation Position (page 37), edge one foot forwards and the other foot back by equal degrees. The heel of one foot will be roughly in line with the toes of the other.

Static Standing Lunge

Another relatively new position for Pilates but it is a position used a lot in gyms. No apologies, Joseph Pilates borrowed from lots of other methods and techniques including yoga, martial arts and ballet. Just remember to apply the ABCs.

A Lunge is normally dynamic but for some exercises in the Pilates Express® programme we are going to use it as a Static Starting Position. Avoid this position if you have knee problems.

01/ Stand tall, feet hip-width apart and parallel.

02/ Step forwards with your right foot, bending the right knee and right hip to about 90 degrees, while simultaneously bending the left knee to as near to parallel as possible. Stay as upright as you can. Because you are 'holding' this Lunge it challenges both your balance and stability.

03/ Return to Starting Position, then repeat bringing the left foot forwards.

WATCHPOINTS

• Step out as far as you can maintain good alignment, depending on your stability and flexibility.

• Double check that your pelvis and spine stay in neutral. You stay as vertical as possible.

• Front leg: the knee stays above your ankle and in line with your second toe.

• Back leg: knee is bent and back heel lifted.

See also Dynamic Lunges (page 160).

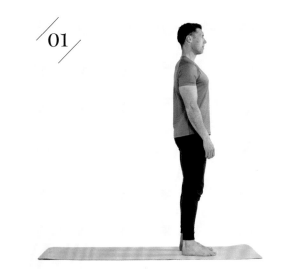

/01/

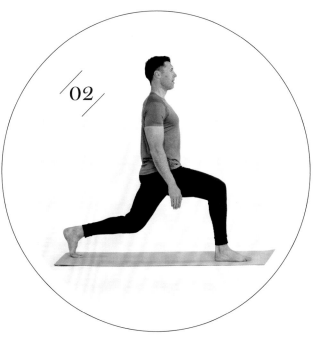

/02/

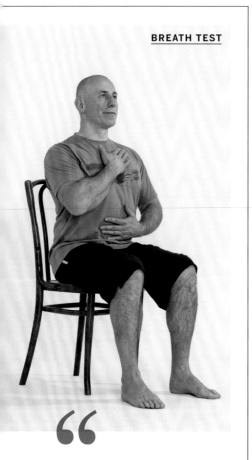

"

*'Breathing
is powerful
medicine.'*

JAMES NESTOR
—— *BREATH*

Breathing

You would have thought that, as we rely so much on oxygen, we would have cracked breathing by now, but most of us still do not breathe efficiently. And yet it is the first thing we do in life and the last... and in between we take approximately 20,000 breaths a day. We take breathing for granted, which is why, if we do struggle to breathe it is so distressing. Asthma sufferers understand this very well, as do those who suffered badly from COVID-19 who reported it was one of the worst symptoms. Long-COVID sufferers complain of breathing difficulties lasting for months. We sincerely hope that the breathing exercises in this book will help you understand and appreciate breathing better.

Just a few minutes of controlled breathing exercises a day can make a huge difference to the quality of your breathing. You can utilise different types of breathing, according to what you are doing or about to do. There are breathing techniques to rejuvenate and refresh, to invigorate or to relax. There are breathing exercises best done in the morning, others in the evening. Some are designed for before exercise, others after. We know that our breathing alters according to our mental state. Knowing how to focus on your breathing and slow your exhalation can be enormously helpful in coping with stressful situations.

As discussed on pages 22-3, the other factor which influences how you breathe is your posture. It is very hard to breathe well if you are hunched. Poor posture means your ribcage and chest are restricted and compressed. Through the Pilates Express® Programme, we hope to get you standing and sitting tall, widening and opening your chest, mobilising your upper spine and ribcage, creating space for you to breathe. And then, we need to give you the strength to maintain this better posture throughout the day. But perhaps we are getting ahead of ourselves. It would be useful to first assess how you are currently breathing.

BREATH TEST

No alcohol required! This simple assessment can be done Seated (page 42–3) or in Relaxation Position (page 37). Notice that in both positions, we ask you to find the right neck alignment. This is very important as the phrenic nerve, which supplies the diaphragm, passes through the C 3, 4, 5 vertebrae of your cervical spine (your neck). Thus, your neck position impacts your breathing.

01/ Sit tall on a sturdy chair, feet hip-width apart and parallel. If you are short, place your feet on a pile of books. Have your weight even on both sitting bones.

02/ Your ribcage should be directly above your pelvis. Lengthen up through the crown of your head; your spine retains its natural curves.

03/ Take a moment to become aware of your neck position; your head should be balanced centrally, floating on top of your spine. Check that your jaw is released.

04/ Place one hand on your chest, the other on your abdomen. (Learn some ways to breathe better on the next page.)

Initially breathe as you would normally. Notice...

• Are you breathing through your nose or mouth?

• Notice where your breath goes. Can you feel your chest lift? Does your breath reach your abdomen? Do your ribs expand sideways?

• Observe your own breathing pattern while you are 'at rest'.

Most of us breathe far too shallowly and much faster than we need to. When this happens, it may limit our supply of oxygen and reduce our ability to eliminate carbon dioxide. If we use mainly the upper part of the chest, we are only using a fraction of our capacity for air. If we breathe more rapidly, we take in a new breath before emptying our lungs of stale air. This stale air is then mixed with the fresh air, decreasing our oxygen supply and therefore our energy.

Your neck alignment affects your breathing

GOOD NECK ALIGNMENT

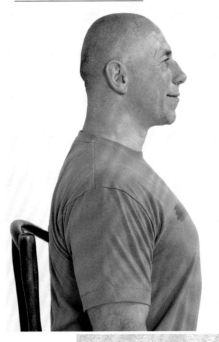

BAD NECK ALIGNMENT

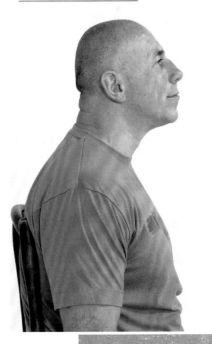

Breathe *better*

Now, let's see if you can improve it. Be kind to yourself here. It will take time to change...

You are going to try to breathe both in and out through your nose. As you take a breath in, allow your breath to travel down low into your abdomen. The hand resting on your chest should stay as still as possible, the hand on your abdomen should rise.

• As you breathe out, reverse the action; emptying from bottom to top.

• Aim for about 8–12 breaths per minute.

You want to focus on a deeper, more rhythmic way of breathing, where the diaphragm is encouraged to move up and down more which, in turn, allows the thoracic cavity to expand fully. A full inhalation followed by a deep exhalation to increase your capacity to inhale fresh air.

Scarf/Band Breathing

This is the traditional way we teach Pilates-style lateral breathing, which is ideal when doing Pilates.

The scarf (or band) gives you sensory feedback so you can feel your ribcage expanding and closing with your breath. Eventually you can practise Scarf Breathing in any of the Starting Positions except Prone, but first try it sitting or standing.

Sit or stand tall and wrap a scarf or stretch band around the lower part of your ribs, crossing it over at the front. If your band is long enough, place the band across the front of your ribcage, then take both ends behind you and cross them over and bring the ends back to the front to hold in each hand. Or tie the band in a knot (not too tight mind!)

With the band wrapped around you like this, you can really feel 360 degrees of the ribcage. If you are comfortable, you could leave the band in place for some of the exercises to remind you to breathe well!

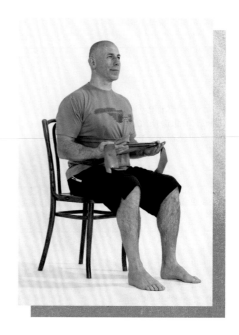

THE EXHALATION

As you breathe out, feel the air gently being pushed out fully as if from the very bottom of your lungs and eventually exiting your body via your nose.

Your diaphragm will begin to rise, and you should feel your ribcage beginning to close as your lungs empty.

THE INHALATION

As you breathe in, visualise balloons swelling gradually with air; your lungs will expand and widen the walls of your ribcage. Do not be tempted to force this inhalation as you will only create tension. You should feel the scarf tightening as your ribs expand.

It is not only the filling up of the lungs that expands your ribcage but also the descent of the diaphragm, lowering into your abdominal area. Therefore, your abdominal area will extend outwards. Try to breathe in through your nose and keep your shoulders relaxed.

Renewed Focus on Your Breathing

There has always been a strong focus on breathing in Pilates, and not just the way we breathe but also the timing, co-ordinating with the movements of each exercise. One of the benefits of Pilates is that you use the breath to facilitate movements and you can reverse that statement too – you can use the movements to facilitate good breathing. For many of the exercises, the timing of your movements will mean that your exhalation is naturally longer than your inhalation. This helps improve your vagal tone (page 15). Remember, you want your breathing to be quiet, rhythmic and controlled.

Turn to Exercises for Respiratory Health (pages 94–121) for more ways to improve your breathing. Reminder: Some people find that focusing too much on their breathing makes them anxious. If this happens, try focusing on other aspects of the exercises – your alignment, centring (see below) and the movements themselves and allow your breath to follow its natural pattern.

Deep Abdominal Breathing for Release

In the next chapter you will learn how to connect to your deep core muscles. This is central to good Pilates practice, but it is very easy to over-engage and overwork these core muscles. It is not just beginners who over-recruit; even experienced Pilates tutors need to learn how to let them go. The easiest way to counter over-recruitment is to spend a few moments practising deep abdominal breathing at the start and end of each workout. When breathing this way, you make use of the piston action of the diaphragm. As you breathe in, the diaphragm descends and there is a corresponding reaction in your pelvic floor; as you breathe out the diaphragm ascends. If you can allow your abdomen to fully expand on the inhalation, this will help to ensure you are not holding onto any unwanted tension.

You can use any position to breathe this way but probably the most successful are Relaxation Position (page 37) and Seated Positions (page 42–3). You can place your hands low on your abdomen to help you. In the Rest Position (page 98), you can simply direct your breath into your abdomen, allowing gravity to assist you. If you suspect you may be over-recruiting your core muscles, spend a few minutes before and/or after your workouts deep abdominal breathing.

SEATED POSITION

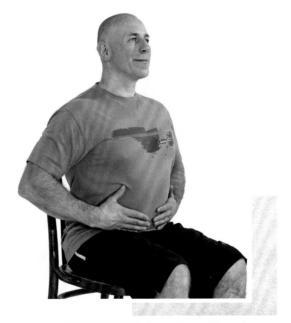

REST POSITION

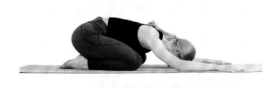

Core Stability and Mobility

In Norse mythology, the god Thor owned a belt 'megingjörd' which, when worn, gave him power and strength.

Sadly, no amount of Pilates, or *Vikings* box sets, will turn us into Norse gods, but, with regular Pilates practice, you can possess your own in-built 'girdle' of strength. How? By working on your Centring.

But what do we mean by Centring? The term encompasses many of the popular and widely talked about concepts associated with 'stability training'. In general terms, we would call an object stable if it can cope with the demands placed on it. For example: a stable chair is built to carry the weight of the person sitting on it and can remain upright if it is, for example, knocked. But stability can also be applied to moving objects – a bicycle can be stable or unstable, for example.

If you are in control of your Alignment and Breathing, then you are probably also Centred. By staying in control of parts that should be moving and keeping still parts that should not, by keeping good alignment of all parts (moving and non-moving!) and by breathing efficiently, you are about there with Centring!

For example, in a Single Knee Fold (page 64), the pelvis needs to be kept still while the leg moves. Whereas in a Spine Curl (page 78), the challenge is to move the spine segmentally, bone by bone, through your midline without tipping the pelvis or spine from side to side or hiking the hip up. Every exercise in Pilates has a stability challenge.

CORE STABILITY

There are many different schools of Pilates. Each has its own way to describe how to engage your core muscles. They include cues such as 'navel to spine', 'use the powerhouse', 'stabilise', 'zip and hollow' – the list goes on. However, the words are not important. What is important is the feeling of the 'connection to inner control' that they try to convey. This connection needs to be found and used as needed to control your movements.

Although much of the stability process is dealt with on a subconscious level, it is also possible to train and improve stability with conscious control. In this section, we will focus on how to find and maintain this connection appropriately. By practising Pilates, we hope to prepare your body so that it will automatically react to any demand placed on it. Your deep core muscles will engage naturally, without prompting. Pilates is based on the principle that by practising control over movements and repeating good movements, you pattern or 'ingrain' these movements into your mind and body, thus improving the quality of your everyday movements.

After all that science, it is good to know too that, while your stability training is helping you to develop a natural corset that wraps around your trunk and supports your spine, it is also streamlining your waistline.

The Dimmer Switch

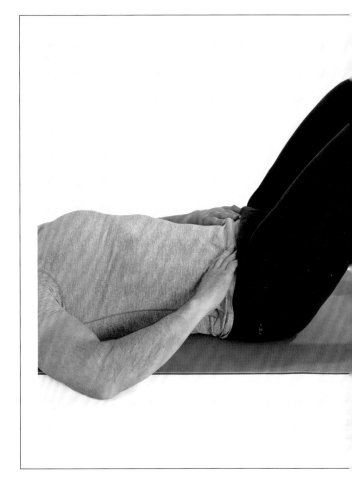

To help remind you of Centring, you will see the following instruction in the exercises:

Use appropriate core connection to control your alignment and movements.

But what do we mean by 'appropriate'? If you were in a class, your teacher would be giving you directions to help you stay stable, but working from a book you will have to figure this out for yourself.

To help, we developed The Dimmer Switch.

As mentioned in the Breathing section (pages 22-5), one of the most common mistakes in Pilates is over-recruitment of the core muscles. The problem is that, if you engage these deep muscles too strongly to begin with, you may end up 'fixing'; becoming rigid, or bracing, and stifling natural movement. The answer is to only engage your deep core as much as you need to control the movement. No more, no less. We call this The Dimmer Switch. Think of adjusting how strongly you use your core muscles as being a little like turning the dial on a dimmer switch up or down.

Thus, you are constantly adjusting the level to match the demands that are placed on the body. If you try the Single and Double Knee Fold (pages 64–5) you will see the amount of centring required relates to the challenge of the exercise being performed. When you try them, notice how you will only need to engage your deep muscles gently for Single Knee Fold, whereas you need to 'turn up the dimmer switch' and engage your core more strongly as you attempt to lift the second leg in Double Knee Fold. As you become proficient at the exercises, you may not need to actively engage your core at all. As you learn to control your alignment through movement, they will automatically engage.

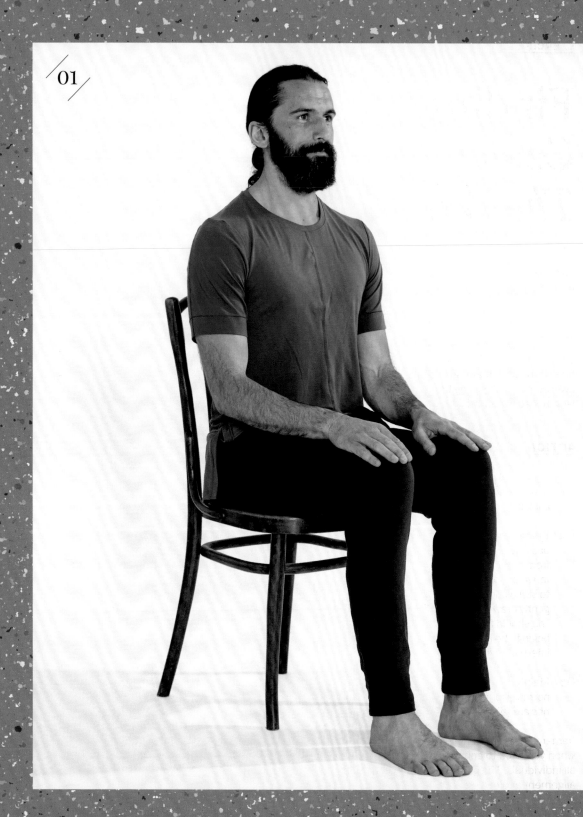

EXERCISE

Finding Your Centre —— *The Wind Zip*

This exercise helps you to feel your deep core muscles and learn how to engage them.

STARTING POSITION

Sit tall on a chair. Place your feet on the floor, hip-width apart. Make sure that your weight is even across both sitting bones and your spine is lengthened in neutral.

ACTION

01/ Take a few moments to breathe deeply, allowing your abomen to expand fully.

02/ Breathe out as you gently squeeze your back passage (anus) as if trying to prevent yourself from passing wind, then bring this feeling forwards towards your pubic bone, as if trying to stop yourself from passing water. Continue to gently draw these pelvic floor muscles up inside. You should feel your abdominals automatically begin to hollow. Imagine you are engaging an internal zip from back to front and up inside.

03/ Maintain this core connection and breathe normally for five breaths. You should feel that your ribs are still free to move. Then relax completely.

Remember The Dimmer Switch and be aware of when you need to engage these muscles. We are all individuals. The goal is to stay in control of your alignment and movements.

WATCHPOINTS

• Ensure that you do not zip, pull up or pull in, too hard. It is very important that you do not force this action or grip.

• Keep your buttocks relaxed and pelvis level. You must not tuck your pelvis under to north.

• Open your chest and the front of your shoulders and avoid any tension in your neck area.

• Keep your breathing smooth and even.

• Your ribcage should expand with your inhalation (a good sign that you haven't over-engaged).

• If you lose any internal connections, relax and start again from the beginning.

• Because you are engaging these pelvic floor muscles from back to front, it makes sense to release them in reverse, front to back.

If identifying your pelvic floor muscles is difficult, try the following (it will come eventually):

• Suck your thumb while drawing up your pelvic floor.

• Stick your tongue out!

• Draw your sitting bones together (this targets another layer of pelvic floor muscles).

• For guys, imagine you are shortening your penis (don't worry, it's not permanent!)

What matters is that you are in control of your body as you move to avoid injury. This will become automatic as you practise more. Try recruiting in different positions; what works for one person, may not work for another.

EXERCISE

Connecting to Your Core

STARTING POSITION

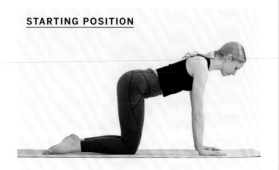

Four-point Kneeling (page 44)

ACTION

01/ Breathe in to prepare.

02/ Breathe out as you gently squeeze your back passage (anus) as if trying to prevent yourself from passing wind, then bring this feeling forwards towards your pubic bone. Draw these muscles up inside until you feel your abdominals automatically begin to hollow.

03/ Maintain this connection and breathe normally for five breaths before releasing, ensuring that your abdominals and ribs are still able to move with your breath.

WATCHPOINTS

• When you engage your core muscles, do not move your spine or pelvis. Later, you will have to move the pelvis and spine!

• Check that you can still breathe easily.

EXERCISE

Challenging Your Centre

Leg Slides, Knee Openings, Single and Double Knee Folds, Knee Fold and Extend

Hopefully by now you are confident about how to place your body in good alignment, breathe laterally and connect to your centre. Now it is time to challenge your ability to control these.

In the following exercises, you will be learning how to move your limbs while keeping your pelvis and spine still, promoting independent movement of your legs at your hip joints. You can vary which exercises you practise each session, but the Starting Position is the same for all of them. Later in the programme, we will be using these exercises repeatedly as ways to challenge you further.

CHALLENGES & BENEFITS

The following pelvic stability exercises (pages 63-67) share similar challenges and benefits, which include:

• Challenge your ability to disassociate the thigh at the hip (move the leg without disturbing your pelvis).

• Challenge your core stability.

• Help ensure safe Pilates practice.

• Mobilise your hips and knees.

• Get your lymph flowing.

Leg Slides

STARTING POSITION

Relaxation Position (page 37), arms lengthened beside you. You can initially place your hands on your pelvis to check for unwanted movement.

ACTION

01/ Breathe in to prepare.

02/ Breathe out as you slide one leg along the floor in line with your hip, keeping your pelvis and spine stable and in neutral.

03/ Breathe in as you draw your leg back in line with your hip to the Starting Position.

Repeat x 5 with each leg.

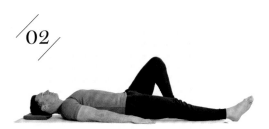

WATCHPOINTS

• Use appropriate core connection to control your alignment and movements.

• Keep your pelvis and spine still and centred throughout. Focus on your leg moving in isolation. Focus on your waist remaining long and even on both sides as you move your leg.

• Keep your foot in contact with the floor and in line with your hip. Keep your chest and front of your shoulders open. Avoid tension in your neck.

• Alternate which leg you start with each time.

Knee Openings

STARTING POSITION

Relaxation Position (page 37) or Seated on a Chair (page 43). Sit towards the front of the chair or, if your seat is square, sit on the corner.

ACTION

01/ Breathe in to prepare.

02/ Breathe out as you allow one knee to slowly open to the side – keep the foot on the mat but allow it to roll to the outer border. Open as far as you can without disturbing the pelvis.

03/ Breathe in as you bring the knee back to the Starting Position.

Repeat x 5 with each leg.

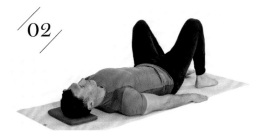

WATCHPOINTS

As for Leg Slides, plus:

• Use appropriate core connection to control your alignment and movements.

• Focus especially on not allowing your pelvis to rock to either side.

• Keep your supporting leg correctly aligned and still; do not allow it to open away from the working leg.

Single Knee Folds

02

STANDING KNEE FOLD

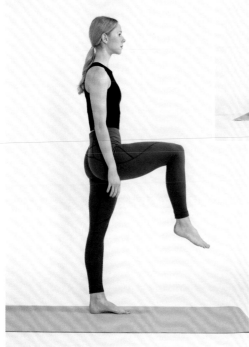

RELAXATION POSITION ACTION

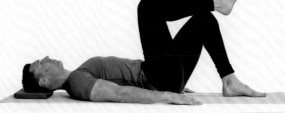

ACTION

01/ Breathe in to prepare.

02/ Breathe out as you fold your knee towards your body.

03/ Breathe in and stay centred.

04/ Breathe out as you slowly return your foot to the mat.

Repeat x 5 with each leg.

WATCHPOINTS

As for Knee Openings, plus:

• Use appropriate core connection to control your alignment and movements.

• Fold your knee in as far as you can without upsetting the pelvis and losing neutral.

• Fold your knee directly in line with your hip joint.

• If Standing, you will need to transfer your weight before you Knee Fold. Focus on lengthening up throughout and keeping both sides of your waist equally long.

• If in Relaxation Position, allow the weight of the leg to drop down into the hip socket. Remain grounded in your pelvis and long in your spine.

Double Knee Folds

We have included Double Knee Folds here because it is a fundamental pelvic stability exercise and will be part of some of the abdominal exercises later. However, it is by no means an easy exercise to perform well and should not be attempted until you are confident performing the previous exercises in this section.

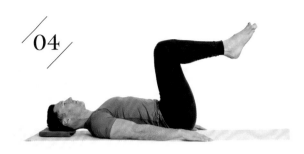

STARTING POSITION

Relaxation Position only (page 37) – do not try this in Standing!

ACTION

01/ Breathe in to prepare.

02/ Breathe out as you fold your right knee in. Remain grounded in your pelvis and long in your spine.

03/ Breathe in and stay centred.

04/ Breathe out as you increase your connection to your centre and fold your left knee towards you.

05/ Breathe in, pelvis grounded in neutral.

06/ Breathe out as you slowly lower your right foot to the mat. Do not allow the abdominals to bulge or your pelvis to lose neutral.

07/ Breathe out as you slowly return the left leg and foot back to the mat.

Repeat x 6, alternating which leg you move first.

WATCHPOINTS

As for Single Knee Folds, plus:

• Bear in mind that lifting and lowering your second knee will require much more stability.

• Continue to breathe!

Moving on... When you are happy that you can do this exercise easily with control, raise and lower each leg, one at a time, but on a single exhalation.

Knee Fold and Extension

A useful preparation for Single Leg Stretch (page 171).

ACTION

Follow Action Points 1–2 above, then:

03/ Breathe in and hold the Knee Fold.

04/ Breathe out as you straighten your leg to an angle of about 45 degrees. Do not disturb your pelvis.

05/ Breathe in and fold the knee in.

06/ Breathe out and lower the foot to the floor with control.

Repeat up to x 8, alternating legs.

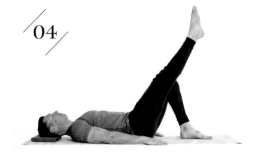

STARTING POSITION

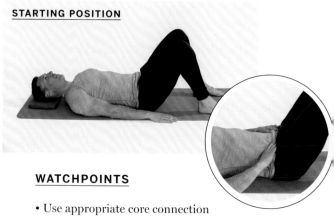

EXERCISE

Knee Rolls

This is a great way to mobilise your hips, whilst challenging your stability and is very useful as a warm-up.

STARTING POSITION

Relaxation Position (page 37) or Seated on a Chair (page 68), see below. Feet slightly wider than hip-width apart. Reach your arms out to the sides slightly lower than shoulder height, palms facing down, or you can place your hands on your pelvis to check for unwanted movement.

ACTION

01/ Breathe in to prepare.

02/ Breathe out as you roll your left leg out from the hip joint and simultaneously roll the right leg in, also from the hip joint. Both knees will roll to the left. Allow your feet to roll too, their borders peeling slightly off the mat.

03/ Breathe out and return both legs back to the centre at the same time.

Repeat on the other side and then repeat the whole sequence up to x 5.

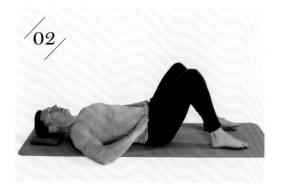

WATCHPOINTS

• Use appropriate core connection to control your alignment and movements.

• Keep your pelvis as still as possible.

• Control the rolling of the knees, do not just let them collapse to one side.

Knee Rolls and Openings

A combination exercise that promotes increased mobility of your hips.

ACTION

Follow Action Points 1–2 above, then:

03/ Breathe in and open your right leg, further 'opening' the hip joint. Stay centred, pelvis as still as possible (it is hard to keep the pelvis completely still).

04/ Breathe out as you roll the right leg inwards.

05/ Breathe in as you roll both legs back to the Starting Position.

Repeat rolling the legs to the other side. Repeat up to 5 times each way.

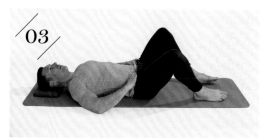

Knee Rolls, Knee openings and Zig Zags

The exercise that keeps on giving... this one feels great, especially if you are feeling tight around the hips. I think of all the new exercises in the book, this is my favourite!

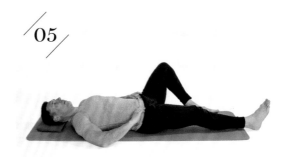

ACTION

Follow Action Points 1–3 from Knee Rolls and Openings, then:

04/ With the leg still turned out, breathe out as you slide it along the floor.

05/ Breathe in and roll the leg in from the hip.

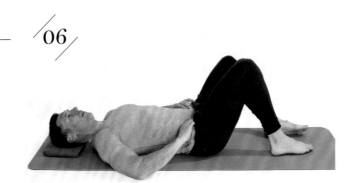

06/ Breathe out as you slide the leg back.

07/ Breathe in and roll both legs back across to the other side.

Repeat both ways up to x 6.

CHALLENGES & BENEFITS

As on page 62.

WATCHPOINTS

As above, plus:

• Try to keep the turn out and the turn in while the leg is sliding.

Moving on... Try all the above exercises (pages 62-67) with your arms lifted – this removes your ability to cheat by stabilising with your arms!

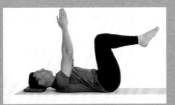
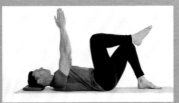

Seated Knee Rolls, Knee Openings and Zig Zags

This is not the best position for this exercise by any means, but if you are stuck in a chair, you will be grateful for the chance to get your hips moving.

Sit tall at the front of a sturdy chair. If the seat of your chair is square, you could sit on the corner to give your hips more space. You will also need to be able to slide your feet easily, so you might have to slip your shoes off. Then you can follow the directions on page 67, taking care that your weight stays even on both sitting bones and you continue to lengthen up through the spine.

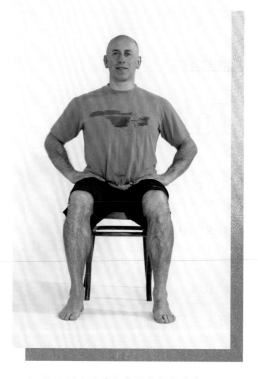

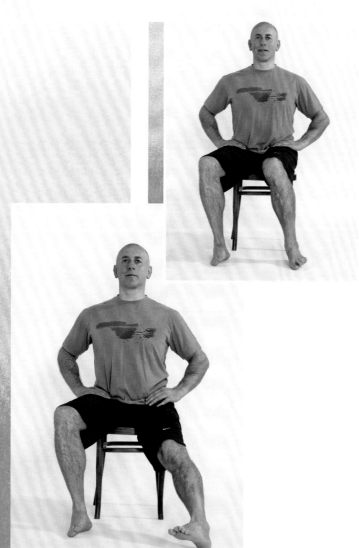

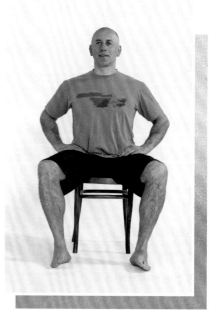

EXERCISE

Table Top

We have broken this important exercise down into stages for you to layer up – you will find some fun variations later (page 144).

STARTING POSITION

Four-point Kneeling (page 44).

ACTION

01/ Breathe in to prepare.

02/ Breathe out as you slide one leg behind you, directly in line with your hip. Your softly pointed foot should remain in contact with the mat. Do not disturb the pelvis or spine.

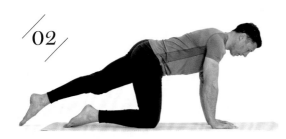

03/ Breathe in and slide the leg back to the Starting Position.

Repeat with the other leg.

Moving on... Follow Action Points 1–2 above, then:

03/ Breathe in as you lengthen and lift your leg to hip height, without moving anything else.

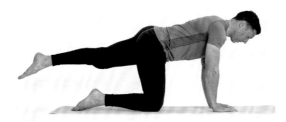

04/ Breathe out and return the foot to the floor and slide it back in.

Repeat with the other leg.

Moving on again... Follow Action Points 1–2 above, then:

03/ Breathe in as you lift the leg to hip height, simultaneously raising the opposite arm forwards, ideally to shoulder height. Maintain a lengthened and stable torso.

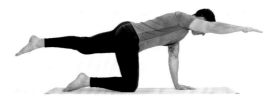

04/ Breathe out and lower your lengthened leg to the mat, simultaneously returning your arm underneath your shoulder.

05/ Breathe in and slide your leg back to the Starting Position.

Repeat up to x 5 on each side, alternating opposite arm and leg.

CHALLENGES & BENEFITS

- Challenges core stability, balance and co-ordination.
- Works your arms, especially the wrists, shoulders, abdominal and gluteal muscles.
- Encourages lymph flow.
- Improves endurance in deep postural muscles.
- Teaches awareness and control of good alignment.

WATCHPOINTS

- Use appropriate core connection to control your alignment and movements.

Oyster

A really valuable, if not particularly popular, exercise! Make sure you take time to line yourself up correctly.

STARTING POSITION

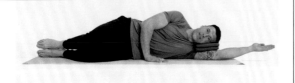

Lie on your left side, in a straight line. Lengthen your left arm underneath your head and in line with your spine – you might need a flat cushion. Have your right hand in front of your ribcage. Bend both knees, with your feet drawn back, so that your heels are aligned with the back of your pelvis. (Place the pillow between your knees, if you wish.)

ACTION

01/ Breathe in to prepare.

02/ Breathe out as you open your top knee, keeping your feet connected. This 'turn out' movement comes from your hip joint. Keep your pelvis still and stable.

03/ Breathe in and, with control, return your leg to the Starting Position.

Repeat up to x 10, then repeat on the other side.

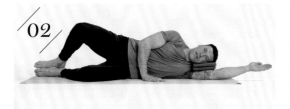

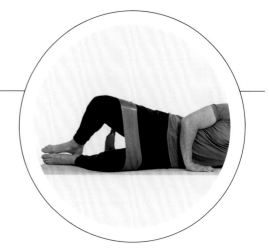

Oyster with Band

Use a stretch band (or a stretchy scarf). Tie it around your thighs. If you are using a scarf do not tie it too tight, just enough to offer resistance, making you work harder!

CHALLENGES & BENEFITS

• Challenges your spinal and pelvic stability.

• Mobilises your hip joint.

• Works your waist and deep gluteal muscles.

• Gets the lymph flowing.

WATCHPOINTS

• Use appropriate core connection to control your alignment and movements.

• Stay aligned, shoulder above shoulder, hip above hip and knee above knee.

• Move your top leg only as far as you can without disturbing the position of your pelvis and spine.

• Keep lengthening both sides of your waist throughout.

• The top arm is positioned to help support you. However, avoid placing too much weight onto it.

• Keep your chest open and your focus directly ahead of you.

EXERCISE

Hip Hinge

This is going to be an important exercise in your Sit to Stand, Stand to Sit Workouts (pages 192–3). It is also an essential part of Squatting (page 150). We want the movement to come from the hips, not the spine, which should stay lengthened and move as one unit. Sounds strange, but imagine that you have swallowed a long stick!

STARTING POSITION

Sit on a sturdy chair, feet hip-width apart and parallel. You will need to be nearer the front of the chair. Place your hands, palms down, in the crease where your legs meet your pelvis.

ACTION

01/ Breathe in to prepare.

02/ Breathe out and, keeping the spine straight (but still with its natural curves), hinge forwards from this crease. The spine moves as one long unit.

03/ Breathe in as you hinge back to upright.

Repeat up to x 5.

CHALLENGES & BENEFITS

- Challenges your ability to align your head, ribcage, spine and pelvis.

- Challenges your ability to disassociate at the hip, isolating trunk and leg movements.

- Mobilises your hips.

STARTING POSITION

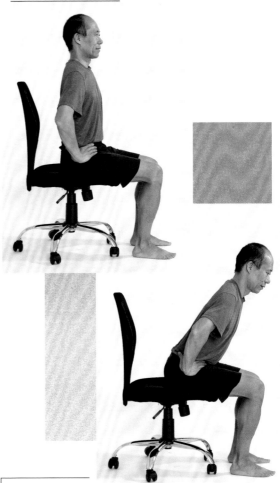

WATCHPOINTS

- Use appropriate core connection to control your alignment and movements.

- You should end up with your **Nose over your Toes**. This will be vital when we use the Hip Hinge as part of Sit to Stand (page 190).

- Take care not to tip your head back or drop it. The back of the neck remains lengthened.

- Check that you are moving solely from the hips, not rounding or arching your back.

- Keeping lengthening through the spine; top and bottom ends!

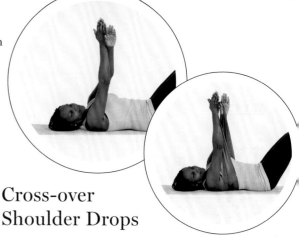

EXERCISE

Shoulder Drops

So far in The New Fundamentals, we have been challenging your core control primarily with the lower limbs, so let's try now with the upper limbs. But before we do, we need to get your shoulders in the best place with Shoulder Drops.

STARTING POSITION

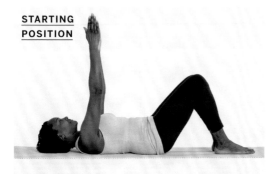

Relaxation Position (page 37). Raise both arms vertically above your chest, shoulder-width apart, palms facing one another.

ACTION

01/ Breathe in as you reach one arm up towards the ceiling, peeling the shoulder blade away from the mat.

02/ Breathe out as you gently release the arm back down, returning the shoulder blade to the mat.

Repeat up to x 10, alternating arms.

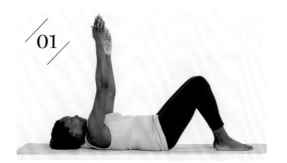

Cross-over Shoulder Drops

Follow the directions above, but instead of reaching straight up with your arm, reach across to the opposite corner of the room. Your head, neck and upper body will rotate with you but keep your pelvis still. You will need to control the release.

Both versions of Shoulder Drops are fabulous done lying on a stretch band as the recoil of the band really helps to release tension. Place the band across your mat so that it is just below your armpits. Make sure you are lying in the middle of the band and have an even amount of band for each arm.

CHALLENGES & BENEFITS

• Challenges your awareness of the position of your shoulders.

• Releases tension from shoulders and neck.

• Gets the lymph flowing.

• If you are doing the cross-over version, you are also mobilising the ribcage and upper spine, helping promote good breathing.

WATCHPOINTS

• Use appropriate core connection to control your alignment and movements.

• Keep your pelvis and spine stable and still.

• Keep your neck long and free from tension; your head remains still and heavy throughout.

• Fully lengthen your arms but avoid locking your elbows.

EXERCISE

Ribcage Closure

A useful exercise that teaches a very important movement skill. We will be revisiting Ribcage Closure in combination with other exercises later.

STARTING POSITION

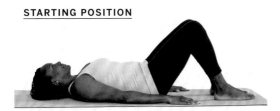

Relaxation Position (page 37). Arms lengthened down by your sides, palms facing inwards (or down.) Take a moment to notice the weight of your ribs, pelvis and head on the mat – this should not change during the exercise. This exercise may also be done in any upright position, although if seated on the mat you will need to start with your arms out in front of your shoulders.

ACTION

01/ Breathe in and raise both arms to shoulder height.

02/ Breathe out as you reach both arms overhead toward the floor. Keep your neck long and encourage the closing of the ribcage. Keep your spine still and stable.

03/ Breathe in as you return the arms above your chest. Feel your ribcage heavy and your collarbones open.

04/ Breathe out and lower your arms, lengthening as you return them by your sides.

Repeat up to x 10.

CHALLENGES & BENEFITS

• Challenges your ability to control the relationship between your arms, ribcage and upper spine.

• Mobilises your shoulders.

• Gets the lymph flowing.

WATCHPOINTS

• Use appropriate core connection to control your alignment and movements.

• Take your arms back to ear level, not to the floor.

• Be particularly careful not to allow your upper spine to arch as you reach your arms overhead.

• Try not to hunch your shoulders; allow them to move naturally and without tension.

• Do not 'fix' the ribcage.

• Fully lengthen your arms but avoid locking elbows.

01/

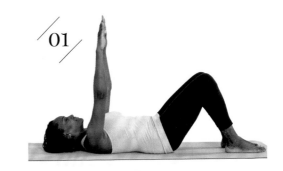

02/

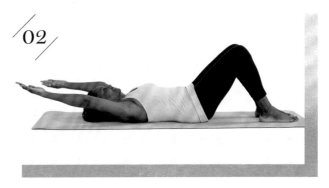

EXERCISE

Single Floating Arms

This exercise is similar to Angel Wings on page 100, but here we want you to focus on the correct order of arm, shoulder blade and collarbone lifting (scapulohumeral rhythm). This action will feature a lot in the standing exercises, for example in a Side Reach (page 89). You can use the skills you learn here whenever you raise your arms in an exercise. Many of us overuse the upper part of our shoulders, which is why these muscles can get really tense. This exercise helps you find a way of lifting your arm that does not overuse these muscles.

As you raise your arm, think of this order of movement: arm, shoulder blade, collarbone. First, just your arm moves up and out, then you will feel the shoulder blade start to coil down and around the back of the ribcage. Finally, the collarbone (clavicle) rises up. With good movement, the shoulder blade will move in the same way as the ballast on a car park security barrier.

ACTION

01/ Breathe in to lengthen up through your spine.

02/ Breathe out as you slowly begin to raise one arm, reaching wide out of the shoulder blades like a bird's wing. Think of the little finger as leading the arm – the arm following the hand as it floats outwards. Keep your arm just in front of your shoulders so that it remains within your peripheral vision. Allow the arm to rotate naturally within the shoulder socket as it lifts.

03/ Breathe in as you lower the arm to your side, following the same pathway.

Repeat x 3 with each arm.

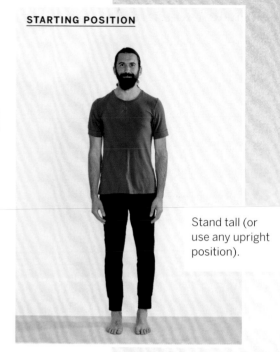

STARTING POSITION

Stand tall (or use any upright position).

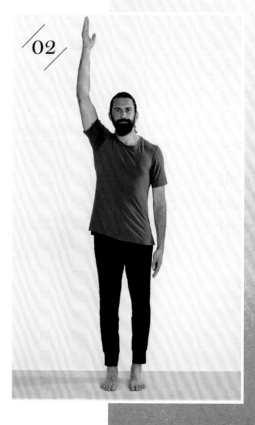

/02/

Double Floating Arms

Simply float both arms up simultaneously.

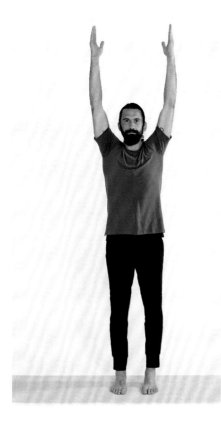

CHALLENGES & BENEFITS

As for Ribcage Closure, plus:

• Challenges core stability.

• Teaches good scapulohumeral rhythm.

WATCHPOINTS

• Use appropriate core connection to control your alignment and movements.

• Add an extra breath, if you need to, at the top of the movement.

• Do not allow your upper body to shift to the side; keep centred.

• Keep the distance between your ears and shoulders but allow the shoulder blade to move.

• Keep your pelvis and spine in neutral.

Single and Double Floating Arms with Weights

For added tone, use hand weights, but not heavy ones or you risk missing the correct sequencing. For a change, as the arms return down, try turning the palms to face down. This gives a wonderful sense of growing up through the crown of the head... think swan rather than duck.

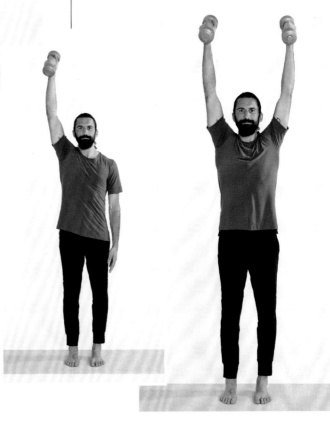

EXERCISE

Arm Circles

A feel-good exercise; great on its own, but even better combined with other movements.

STARTING POSITION

Relaxation Position (page 37), or any upright position. It can also be added to different exercises, such as Standing Back Bends (as shown opposite), Spine Curls (page 78) or Hip Rolls (page 88).

ACTION

01/ Breathe in to prepare.

02/ Breathe out as you raise both arms overhead towards the floor, without disturbing your spine, ribcage or pelvis.

03/ Breathe in as you circle your arms out to the sides and down towards your body. Once your arms are below shoulder height, turn the palms to the mat and return the arms to the Starting Position.

Repeat x 5, then reverse the direction.

CHALLENGES & BENEFITS

• Challenges your ability to move your arms freely, with control and without overuse of upper shoulder muscles.

• Mobilises the shoulders.

• Gets the lymph flowing.

• If you do Arm Circles in a Standing position with a Squat (page 150) or Dynamic Lunge (page 160), it can help add an aerobic element to your workout, getting your heart pumping.

WATCHPOINTS

• Use appropriate core connection to control your alignment and movements.

• Enjoy the free movement of your arms and shoulders but try to keep your ribcage connected down towards your waist and upper spine still.

• Remember what you learnt in Floating Arms – the arms move first and then, as they reach overhead, allow the shoulder blades to glide smoothly around the ribcage.

• As the arms circle, keep them on the same level.

• If you use an upright position, and your flexibility permits, you can take your arms slightly behind you as they descend past your shoulders to circle down and round.

STARTING POSITION

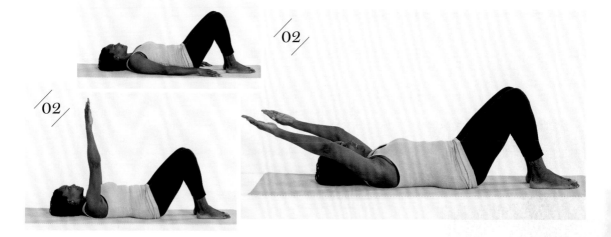

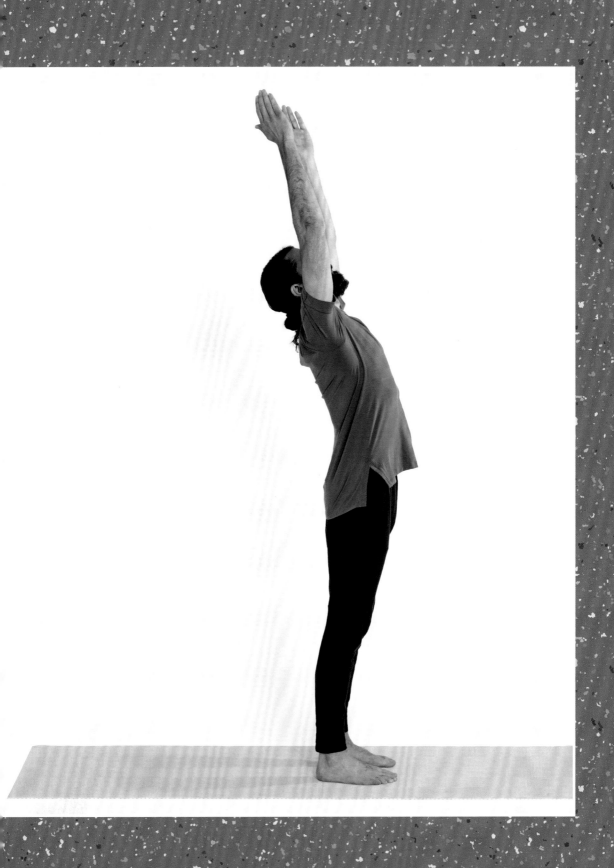

EXERCISE

Mobility

As mentioned, stability is not about being still, you need to be stable when you move too. Thus, we need to challenge your stability through every plane of movement as every day we need to bend, twist, lift, squat, climb…

For any workout to be balanced, it needs to include all the spinal movements: flexion (bending forwards); rotation (twisting); side flexion (side bending) and extension (bending backwards).

Spine Curls

A personal favourite, this popular exercise is a great warm-up, hence you will find it in most of the mat mini workouts. Axial length through your Centreline is all-important.

STARTING POSITION

Relaxation Position (page 37), arms lengthened down the sides of your body, palms down.

ACTION

01/ Breathe in to prepare.

02/ Breathe out as you curl your tailbone under, tilting the pelvis to north and then peel your spine off the mat one vertebra at a time, lengthening your knees away from your hips. Roll your spine sequentially, bone by bone, to the tips of the shoulder blades.

03/ Breathe in and hold this position, focusing on the length in your spine.

04/ Breathe out as you roll the spine back down, softening the breastbone and wheeling each bone down in turn.

05/ Breathe in as you release the pelvis back to level again.

Repeat up to x 10.

STARTING POSITION

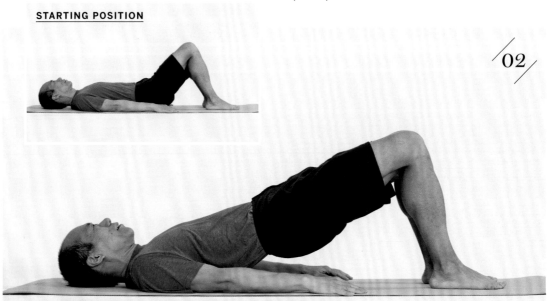

/02/

CHALLENGES & BENEFITS

• Challenges your ability to articulate the spine segmentally bone by bone, as opposed to in chunks!

• Challenges your spatial awareness; can you land the spine centrally, not tipping to one side?

• Mobilises your spine and hips.

• Works your gluteal muscles and abdominals.

WATCHPOINTS

• Use appropriate core connection to control your alignment and movements.

• Roll through your Centreline.

• Keep equal weight through both feet to avoid your pelvis dipping to either side.

• Keep the waist equally long on both sides, knees parallel, in line with your hips, and avoid your feet rolling in or out.

Split Stance Spine Curls

Following the directions opposite but with your feet in a staggered position. This will increase the challenge to roll the spine through your Centreline.

Start in Relaxation Position (page 37) but move one foot forward a few inches and one foot back. Spine Curl as before but focus not just on rolling through the spine but also on keeping to your Centreline. The challenge is not to allow the pelvis or spine to dip to one side as you roll.

Repeat up to x 3, then swap the feet to repeat on the other side.

Moving on... You can add a wide variety of arm actions to Spine Curls, such as Ribcage Closure (page 73) or Arm Circles (page 76). When doing this, always try to time it so that your arms return to the Starting Position as your tailbone lands and your pelvis is back in neutral.

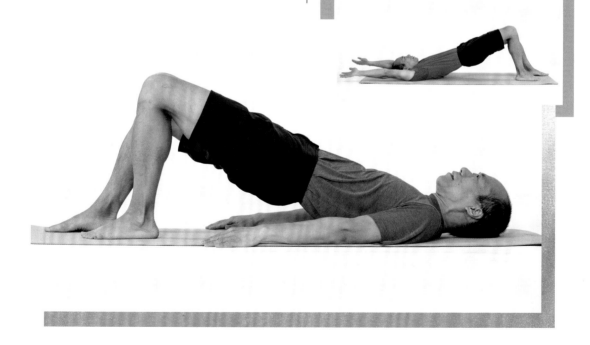

EXERCISE

Cat

A great way to keep your spine flexible. You will need to create the shape of an elongated C-Curve in this exercise and, also, a reverse C-Curve, which takes you into a gentle back extension.

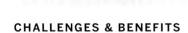

/02/

/04/

STARTING POSITION

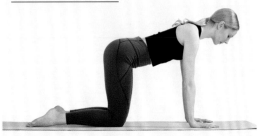

Four-point Kneeling (page 44), although we will also show you other positions such as Seated (page 42–3) and Standing (page 50).

ACTION

01/ Breathe in and lengthen your spine.

02/ Breathe out as you roll your pelvis underneath you, as if directing your tailbone between your legs. Your lower back will gently round and then your upper back, followed by your neck, and finally nod your head slightly forwards to create a long C-Curve.

03/ Breathe in wide.

04/ Breathe out as you simultaneously start to unravel the spine, sending the tailbone away from the crown of your head, gently extending the entire spine into a reverse C-Curve. Shine your breastbone forwards, collarbones wide and open.

05/ Breathe in and return to neutral.

CHALLENGES & BENEFITS

• Challenges your ability to flex and extend the spine smoothly, articulating bone by bone.

• Challenges your proprioception (awareness of joint positions.

• Mobilises your spine and hips.

• Promotes flexibility in spine and ribcage.

• Helps back breathing by encouraging mobility of the intercostal muscles between the ribs.

WATCHPOINTS

• Use appropriate core connection to control your alignment and movements.

• Aim for even, elongated C-Curves. A common mistake is to overly round the upper back in C-Curve and overly dip in the low back in reverse C-Curve.

• Keep the head following the same curved line of the spine; do not drop it down too far.

• Keep the weight evenly distributed between both hands and knees.

• Fully lengthen your arms but avoid locking your elbows.

One-armed Cat

This works your arms and shoulders, as well as challenging your core. The challenge is to move the spine as centrally as you can. You may not achieve much back extension with this version.

Starting Position as before, but this time, wrap one arm around your ribs.

Repeat x 3 with each arm.

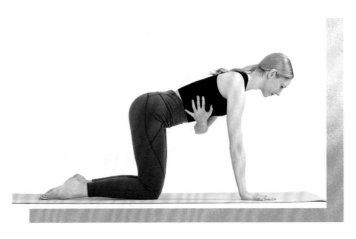

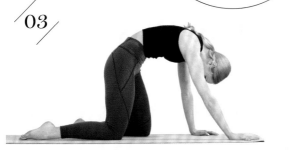

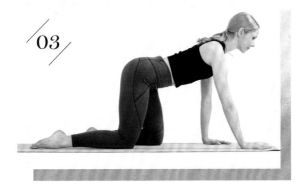

Split Stance Cat

There are a variety of ways you can apply the Split Stance to Cat. You could:

01/ Stagger the arms.

02/ Stagger the knees.

03/ Stagger both knees and arms; right knee forwards, right hand forwards or right knee forwards, left hand forwards.

Follow all the directions for Cat. Repeat x 3, then swap which knee/arm is in front.

Remember, the challenge here, in addition to those already mentioned, is to curl and unfurl the spine, lengthening through the Centreline, and trying to resist unwanted rotation.

Seated Cat

It is great that Cat can be done in a variety of positions. Sitting is not the best option as it is not as easy to roll your tailbone under but, if you are stuck at your desk, it is a good way to mobilise the spine and hips.

STARTING POSITION

Sit tall in the centre of a sturdy chair, feet hip-width apart. Place your hands lightly on top of your thighs.

ACTION

01/ Breathe in to lengthen the spine.

02/ Breathe out as you roll your tailbone under, curling the spine forwards into an elongated C-Curve.

03/ Breathe in and hold the position.

04/ Breathe out as you roll the pelvis forwards, sticking out your sitting bones and lifting the spine up into extension, shining your breastbone forwards and up.

05/ Breathe in and hold the position.

06/ Breathe out and roll the tailbone under again to repeat.

Repeat up to x 6, before coming back to sit tall.

CHALLENGES & BENEFITS

As for Cat, plus:

• Challenge your ability to elongate the spine while seated.

WATCHPOINTS

• Use appropriate core connection to control your alignment and movements.

• Keep the weight even on both sitting bones throughout.

• Try to keep the C-Curve even throughout the length of the spine; do not over-round or arch any one section. The end position should be as for C-Curve above.

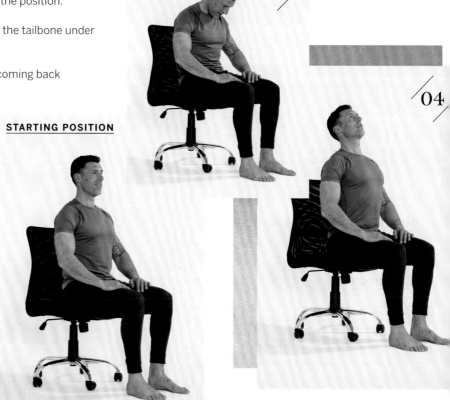

STARTING POSITION

Standing Cat

Incredibly useful for when you cannot use your mat. The Standing position also enables you to roll through your hips better.

STARTING POSITION

Stand tall, feet hip's width apart, then hinge forwards into a Squat (page 150). Place your hands on your thighs. Have your elbows slightly bent, elbows and collarbones wide.

ACTION

01/ Breathe in to lengthen your spine.

02/ Breathe out and roll your tailbone under, curling the spine into an elongated C-Curve.

03/ Breathe in and hold the position.

04/ Breathe out and send your tailbone away from the crown of your head, pelvis moving into an anterior tilt and then lifting segmentally up through the spine, bone by bone, into extension.

05/ Breathe in and hold the position.

06/ Breathe out and curl the tailbone under.

Repeat up to x 6 before coming back into a neutral spinal position and then hinging back upright with control.

VARIATION:

You can either move segmentally through the spine from top to bottom or from bottom to top, or you can move top end and bottom end simultaneously.

CHALLENGES & BENEFITS

As for Cat and Squats!

WATCHPOINTS

As for Cat and Squats.

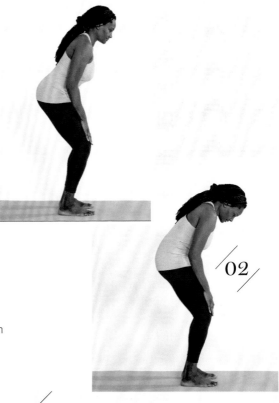

/02/

/04/

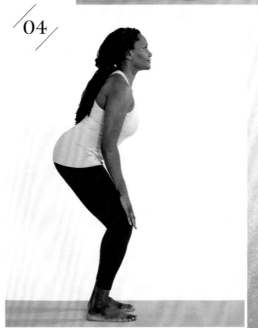

EXERCISE

Curl Ups

This is such a common exercise that it is easy to forget that, done properly, with control, it is one of the best abdominal exercises ever. Pay close attention to the detail or you will miss out on the benefits.

ACTION

01/ Breathe in to prepare.

02/ Breathe out as you lengthen the back of your neck, nod your head and sequentially curl up the upper body, keeping the back of your lower ribcage in contact with the mat. Keep your pelvis still and level and do not allow your abdominals to bulge.

03/ Breathe into the back of your ribcage and maintain this curled-up position.

04/ Breathe out as you slowly and sequentially roll the spine back down to the mat with control.

Repeat up to x 10.

STARTING POSITION

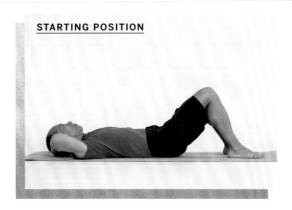

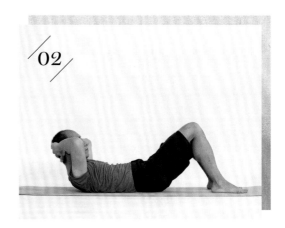

Relaxation Position (page 37). Float both arms to lightly clasp behind your head, ensuring that, as you do so, you do not arch your upper back. Have your elbows open and positioned just in front of your ears, within your peripheral vision.

WATCHPOINTS

• Use appropriate core connection to control your alignment and movements.

• Pelvis remains in neutral throughout; curl up only as far as this can be maintained.

• Focus on wheeling your spine off the mat, vertebra by vertebra.

• Control the sequential return of your spine back down to the mat.

• Add an extra breath to curl up higher, if you wish.

CHALLENGES & BENEFITS

• Challenges your ability to control trunk flexion sequentially, while keeping the pelvis stable.

• Mobilises the upper spine and helps to improve breathing.

• Works the abdominals.

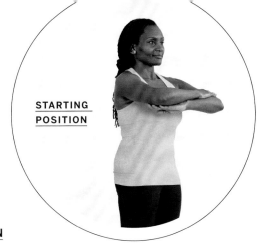

EXERCISE

Waist Twist

The muscles that help you twist are the very same ones that define your waist. As with all our exercises, lengthen up through the crown of the head and spiral up, up and up as you rotate around your central axis, visualizing your Centreline.

ACTION

01/ Breathe in and lengthen up through your spine.

02/ Breathe out as you move your gaze to the right; turning your head, then neck and finally rotating your torso fully to the right. Keep your pelvis still and keep lengthening up through the crown of the head.

03/ Breathe in as you continue to lengthen your spine and rotate back to the Starting Position.

Repeat x 6 to each side. After three turns, change your arm position so that the underneath arm is now on top.

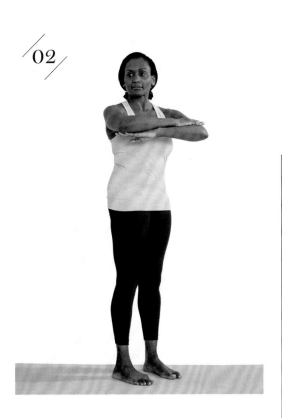

/02/

This exercise can be done in any upright position. We will try Standing here (page 50).

Stand tall, legs in parallel, hip-width apart. Fold your arms in front of your chest, just below shoulder height. One palm is on top of the opposite elbow and the other hand is positioned underneath the opposite elbow.

CHALLENGES & BENEFITS

- Challenges you to achieve axial length and segmental rotation of the upper and mid-spine around your Centreline, while keeping the pelvis still.

- Mobilises the upper spine and thus helps promote better breathing.

WATCHPOINTS

- Use appropriate core connection to control your alignment and movements.

- Your pelvis should remain still. Keep the weight even on both feet (or on both sitting bones if you are seated, both knees if High Kneeling; page 46) and maintain their contact with the mat/floor throughout.

- Avoid arching your back or shortening your waist.

- Carry your arms with the spine; do not allow them to lead the movement.

EXERCISE

Bow *and* Arrow

A feel-good rotation exercise that can also be done in a variety of positions. We have given you Side Lying (page 49) and Standing (page 50) here, but you will also find Bow and Arrow in other upright positions in the workouts (page 178).

Side-lying Bow and Arrow

STARTING POSITION

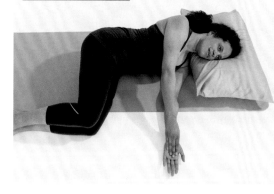

Side Lying on the left. Place a substantial cushion (a bed pillow works fine) underneath your head to ensure that your head and neck are in line with your spine. Bend both knees in front of you so that your hips and knees are bent to a right angle. Place another pillow between your knees if you wish. Lengthen both arms out in front of your body at shoulder height.

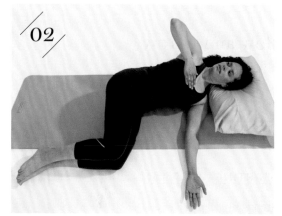

/02/

ACTION

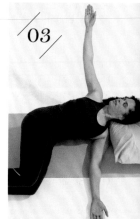

/03/

01/ Breathe in to prepare.

02/ Breathe out as you bend your right elbow, drawing the arm towards your body and right hand towards the shoulder. Simultaneously, rotate your head, neck and upper spine (in that order) to the right.

03/ Breathe in as you straighten the arm while continuing to lengthen the spine and encouraging a little more rotation.

04/ Breathe out as you rotate your spine back to the Starting Position, keeping the arm straight.

Repeat up to x 5 to each side.

CHALLENGES & BENEFITS

• Challenges your ability to rotate segmentally with axial length.

• Challenges your co-ordination and control of alignment in Side Lying.

• Mobilises your spine, shoulders and elbows.

• Works your waist.

Bow and Arrow ———
Standing or Seated

The arm action and spinal rotation are the same. You may find it more challenging in these upright positions.

STARTING POSITION

Stand tall or sit tall. If Standing (page 50), check your weight is even on both feet. If Seated (page 42–3), ensure the weight is even across both your sitting bones.

In either position, your arms are lengthened in front you, slightly lower than shoulder height and shoulder-width apart. The arms are parallel, palms facing down.

ACTION

01/ Breathe in to prepare.

02/ Breathe out as you bend your right elbow, drawing the arm towards your body and right hand towards the shoulder. Simultaneously, rotate your head, neck and upper spine (in that order) to the right.

03/ Breathe in as you straighten the arm while lengthening the spine and encouraging a little more rotation.

04/ Breathe out as you rotate your spine back to the Starting Position, keeping the arm straight.

Repeat x 5 to each side.

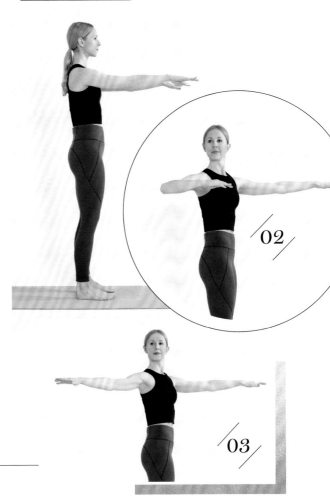

WATCHPOINTS

• Use appropriate core connection to control your alignment and movements.

• Visualise your Centreline. Rotate with length around it.

• Keep spiralling up, up, up as you twist.

• Both sides of your waist remain equally long. If Side Lying, you will need to keep checking your waist is lifted, this will help you keep your Centreline.

• Your arm stops moving when your spine stops moving; do not be tempted to open it further.

EXERCISE

Hip Rolls

Another fabulous rotation exercise, which you
can combine with other movements (pages 110-11).

STARTING POSITION

Relaxation Position (page 37). Bring your feet and legs together
and connect your inner thighs. Reach your arms out on the mat
slightly lower than shoulder height, palms facing up.

ACTION

01/ Breathe in to prepare.

02/ Breathe out as you roll your pelvis to the left (like rolling
east in Compass, page 38). The right side of the pelvis and
the lower right ribs will peel slightly off the mat.

03/ Breathe in as you return the pelvis and legs back to the
Starting Position, initiating from your centre.

Repeat to the other side and then repeat the whole sequence
up to x 5.

VARIATION:

Rotate your head the opposite way.

CHALLENGES & BENEFITS

• Challenges your ability to
rotate segmentally around your
Centreline with axial length.

• Mobilises your spine.

• Works your waist.

WATCHPOINTS

• Use appropriate core connection
to control your alignment and
movements.

• Roll your pelvis and legs directly
to the side and avoid any detours.

• Keep both sides of your waist
equally long.

• Maintain a connection between
your ribcage and pelvis and
ensure that you don't arch your
back as you roll.

• As you roll, roll first through
your hips, waist and finally
lower ribs, returning lower
ribs, waist and finally hips.

/02/

STARTING POSITION

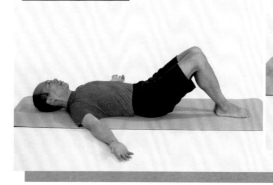

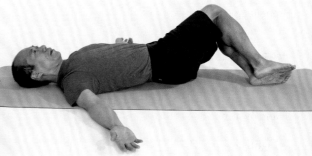

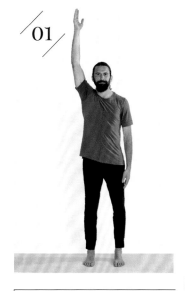

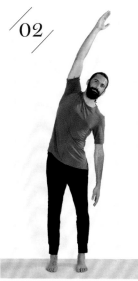

Side Reach

This wonderful exercise both stretches and works the waist.

STARTING POSITION

This exercise can be performed in any upright position (although later in the book, we have also given you versions in prone, when combined with The Dart (page 119) and Relaxation Position (page 102). There is a challenging High Kneeling version on page 162.

Stand tall, legs in parallel and, note, shoulder-width apart. Allow your arms to lengthen down by your sides.

ACTION

01/ Breathe in as you raise your right arm out to the side and overhead.

02/ Breathe out as you reach up and over, leading with your head, sequentially bending your spine to the left.

03/ Breathe into your right ribcage.

04/ Breathe out as you return the spine back to the vertical position. Lower your right arm down by your side.

Repeat up to x 5 to each side.

VARIATIONS:

• Having floated one arm up, lightly clasp your hand behind your head and direct the elbow up and over in a long arc to stretch.

• Lightly clasp both hands behind your head to increase the challenge.

CHALLENGES & BENEFITS

• Challenges you to move the spine segmentally and smoothly into side flexion.

• Challenges your ability to side flex in one plane only without deviation.

• Mobilises your spine and shoulders.

• Opens your ribcage and thus promotes better breathing.

• Tones your waistline.

WATCHPOINTS

• Use appropriate core connection to control your alignment and movements.

• Move in one plane only, avoid curving forwards or arching back.

• Keep your pelvis still and central and head and neck in line with the rest of your spine.

• Keep the weight even on both feet if you are Standing, both sitting bones if you are Seated and both knees if you are High Kneeling.

• It helps to visualise breathing into the open side, then you can use the closing of the ribs to help you return upright.

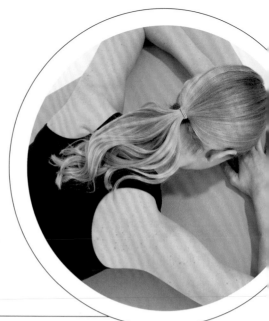

EXERCISE

Diamond Press

It is very easy to forget about your back. We look in the mirror front and side, but very rarely check out the rear view. When I first started Pilates, this was the only back extension exercise I could do with any degree of success. Now, one of my favourite exercises is Full Cobra.

STARTING POSITION

Prone (page 48). Create a diamond shape with the arms, place the fingertips together, palms down onto the mat and open your elbows (you may place the hands wider if it allows your shoulders to broaden more). Rest your forehead on the backs of the hands (or a towel). Your legs are hip-width apart and parallel. If you wish, you may place a folded towel or flat cushion under your abdomen to support your lumbar spine.

ACTION

01/ Breathe in to prepare.

02/ Breathe out as you lift your head, then your neck and then your chest off the mat. Feel your lower ribs remaining in contact with the mat but shine your breastbone forwards, opening your chest. Breathe in as you hold thislengthened and stable position.

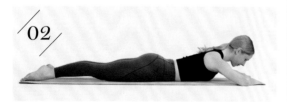

/02/

03/ Breathe out as you lengthen and return your chest, neck and head sequentially back to the Starting Position.

Repeat up to x 8.

CHALLENGES & BENEFITS

• Challenges you to control the segmental extension of your upper spine.

• Mobilises your upper spine to help promote better breathing.

• Helps correct rounded posture.

• Works your back extensors.

WATCHPOINTS

• Use appropriate core connection to control your alignment and movements.

• Grow, grow, grow – think forwards and up.

• Initiate by lengthening and lifting first your head (think of rolling a marble away along the mat with your nose) and then your neck. When your head and neck are in line with your spine, start to extend the upper spine.

• Keep your lower ribs in contact with the mat as you extend. Length is more important than height.

• Keep your feet in contact with the mat throughout.

• As you return to the mat, do not collapse – return with length and control. Remember your Centreline.

EXERCISE

Cobra Prep

Use what you have learnt doing Diamond Press (opposite).

STARTING POSITION

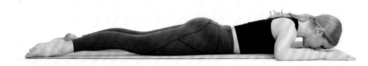

Prone, resting your forehead on the mat (use a folded towel underneath if necessary). Legs straight, slightly wider than hip-width and turned out from the hips. Bend your elbows and position your hands slightly wider than, and just above, shoulder height. Make sure that your shoulders are released and collarbones are wide.

ACTION

01/ Breathe in to prepare.

02/ Breathe out as you begin to lengthen the front of your neck. Roll and lift your head and then chest off the mat. Your lower ribs should remain in contact with the mat, but open your chest and focus on directing it forwards.

03/ Breathe in as you hold this lengthened and lifted position.

04/ Breathe out as you return your chest and head sequentially back down to the mat, allowing the arms to bend back to the Starting Position.

Repeat up to x 8.

CHALLENGES & BENEFITS

- Challenges your ability to extend the upper spine sequentially with control.

- Mobilises the spine.

- Works your back muscles.

- Counters hunched posture.

WATCHPOINTS

- Use appropriate core connection to control your alignment and movements.

- Move smoothly with axial length through your Centreline.

- Keep your legs on the mat, reaching away from you throughout.

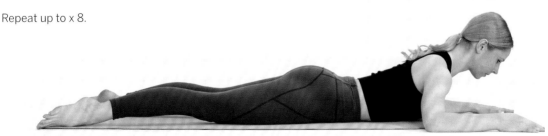

EXERCISE

Standing Back Bend

We will be using this later in the workouts as it is a great option if you are at work or out and about and do not have a mat handy.

STARTING POSITION

Standing tall in parallel, hands relaxed down by your sides or lightly clasped behind your head (this supports your neck). If clasped behind your head, ensure that your elbows remain in your peripheral vision.

ACTION

01/ Breathe in and, initiating with the head, begin to gently bend backwards sequentially, arching the spine evenly, vertebra by vertebra. Aim for an even curve along the whole spine.

02/ Breathe out as you begin to restack the spine sequentially from the bottom to the top, lengthening as you do so.

Repeat up to x 8.

STARTING POSITION

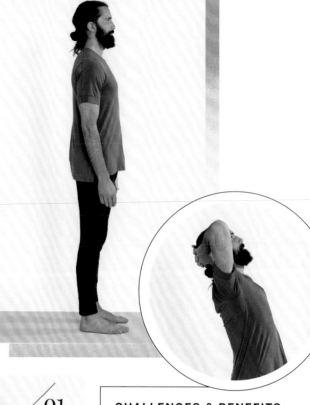

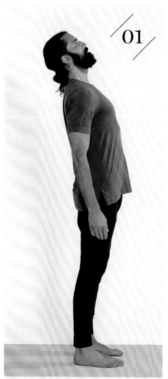

01

CHALLENGES & BENEFITS

• As for Cobra Prep (above), plus you have the additional challenge of maintaining good postural alignment in Standing without the feedback and support of the floor.

WATCHPOINTS

• Use appropriate core connection to control your alignment and movements.

• Move directly with axial length through your Centreline.

• Keep the head following the same curved line of the spine – do not tip it back too far.

• Ground yourself through your feet, keeping the weight even.

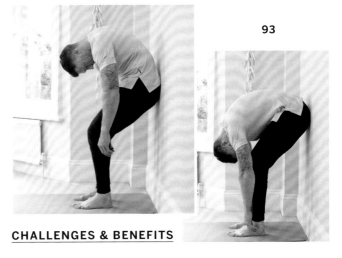

EXERCISE

Roll Downs

Roll Downs are an ideal way to finish a session. It is a good idea to practise against a wall initially before trying the freestanding version.

STARTING POSITION

Stand tall with your back against a wall, feet parallel and hip-width apart, approximately 1–2 feet from the wall with knees slightly bent. Keep the back of your ribcage and pelvis in contact with the wall and your spine should retain its natural curves. The back of your head may, or may not, be in contact depending on your posture. Allow your arms to lengthen down by your sides.

ACTION

01/ Breathe in as you lengthen the back of your neck and nod your head forwards.

02/ Breathe out as you continue to roll your spine forwards and down. Peel each vertebra from the wall in turn until you can wheel no more, then bend forwards from the hips.

03/ Breathe in as you roll your pelvis under and restack the vertebrae, rolling the spine back up the wall.

Repeat up to x 5.

CHALLENGES & BENEFITS

• Challenges your ability to articulate the spine sequentially into flexion and extension.

• Challenges you to move smoothly with axial length through your Centreline.

• Mobilises the spine and hips.

• Works your back muscles.

• Releases tension in the upper body.

WATCHPOINTS

• Use appropriate core connection to control your alignment and movements.

• Roll smoothly and sequentially through each segment of your spine.

• Connect your deep abdominals to support your spine.

• As you roll down, begin the movement with a nod of your head.

• Roll with axial length through your Centreline.

• Keep your weight balanced evenly on both feet.

Freestanding Roll Downs

Apply what you have learnt in Roll Downs against a Wall (above) to this freestanding version. The directions are the same, minus the wall. You'll have to decide how bent your knees should be to allow you to roll comfortably through the spine. This exercise is about mobilising the spine and hips, not stretching the hamstrings. Look out for exercises in the Workouts that require you to heel raise, coming up onto your toes, when you have finished your Roll Downs. Challenging!

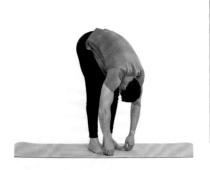

Exercises for *Respiratory* Health

This chapter is full of wonderful exercises for improving your breathing at the same time as working the rest of your body. You will find a mix of controlled breathing exercises and exercises that encourage better breathing by mobilising your upper spine and ribcage.

Remember... Quiet, Controlled, Rhythmic Breathing

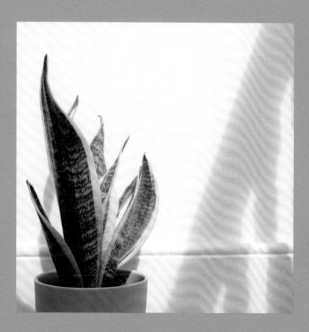

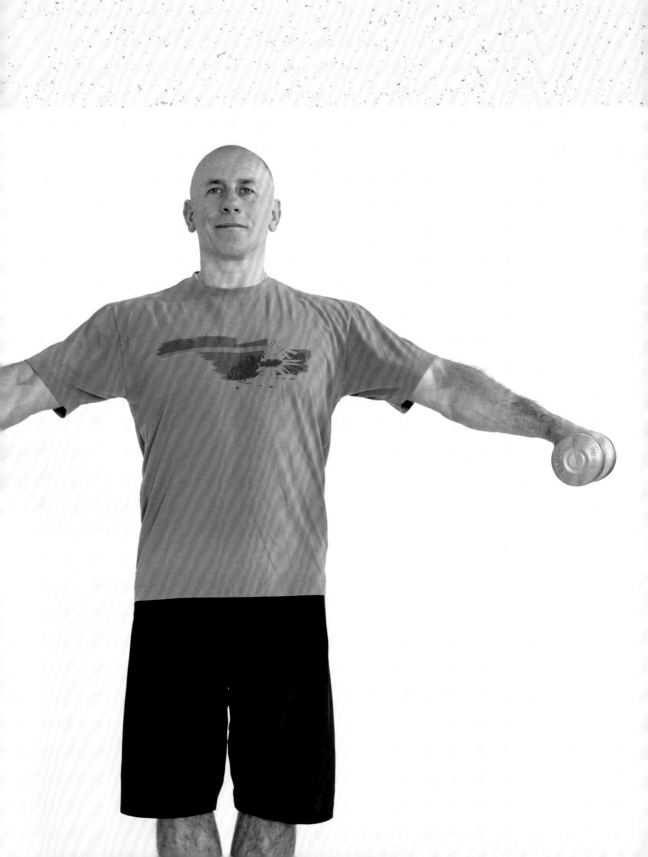

EXERCISE

Box *or* Tactical Breathing

Adapted from an old Navy Seals breathing technique, this simple exercise can be done at any time of day, in any position. The four count creates a 'neutral' state of mind, which means it neither over-calms nor excites. This makes it very practical to do at the bus stop or at your desk. It also means it can be used at the start or end of a Pilates session.

Sit, stand or lie tall! Shoulders relaxed, chest open, spine long, feet grounded. Think of a box, each side is a count of four.

ACTION

01/ Breathe in for a count of four.

02/ Hold your breath for a count of four.

03/ Breathe out for a count of four.

04/ Hold for a count of four.

Repeat for up to 3 minutes maximum.

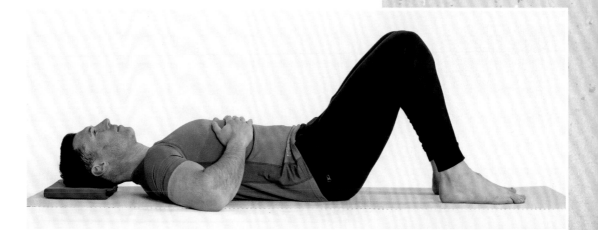

Vagal Tone Breathing

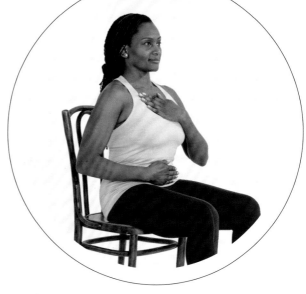

This exercise improves your vagal tone by altering your breathing pattern so your exhalation is longer than your inhalation. You can try this in any position, but we suggest Relaxation Position (page 37) or Seated (page 43), initially, as then you are supported. Place one hand just below your navel, the other on your chest.

ACTION

01/ Breathe in slowly for a count of three, breathing right down into your abdomen, allowing it to fully expand.

02/ Breathe out slowly, to a count of six, if you can manage it; five if not. Empty your lungs fully and completely before breathing in again.

One Lung Breathing

/01/

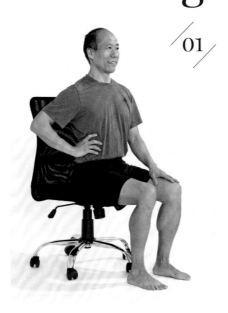

Do not take this title too seriously; you will also be breathing into the other lung! However, it really does help if you are stiff on one side. Add a few extra breaths on your tighter side, if you like.

STARTING POSITION

Stand or sit tall, or lie in Relaxation Position (page 37).

ACTION

01/ Place your right hand on your right rib, fingers at the front, thumb around the back.

02/ Keeping your posture central, without shifting to one side, breathe into the right lung and ribcage. Take five deep breaths, then swap hands and sides and repeat.

Alternate which side you start with first.

EXERCISE

Rest Position — Back Breathing

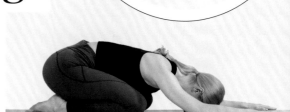

This exercise is used a lot in Pilates after back extension exercises like Dart (page 119), Star (page 146), Diamond Press (page 90) and Cobra (page 170). It is useful as a breathing position because it encourages you to breathe into your back; an area we often find hard to expand. It also provides an opportunity to refocus concentration in preparation for the next exercise.

STARTING POSITION

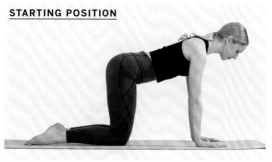

From a prone position, come up into Four-point Kneeling (page 44).

ACTION

01/ Breathe in wide as you bring your feet slightly closer together.

02/ Breathe out as you fold at your hips, directing your buttocks backwards and down. Keep your hands on the mat and lengthen your arms. Ideally (see Watchpoints), rest your sitting bones on your heels, chest on your thighs and forehead on the mat.

03/ Breathe in and direct the breath into the back and sides of your ribs and feel the ribcage progressively expand. Imagine the back of your ribs are like giant fish gills.

04/ Breathe out, fully emptying your lungs and focus on closing the ribs down and together.

Repeat up to x 10.

To finish, breathe out and begin by rolling your pelvis underneath you, then sequentially roll and restack your spine to an upright position, sitting back onto the heels.

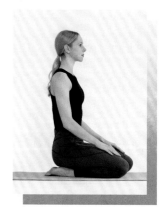

WATCHPOINTS

• Use appropriate core connection to control your alignment and movements.

• Avoid opening your knees too wide; the thighs should be slightly apart and underneath the ribcage.

• Allow your head to be heavy, neck lengthened and relaxed.

• Depending on your flexibility, you may need to rest your head on cushions (or folded hands) and/or you may need cushions under your bottom.

EXERCISE

360 Degrees — Hundred Breathing

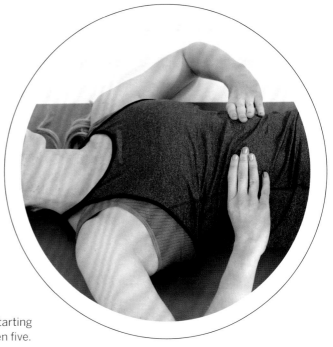

Here we use your hand position to encourage you to expand the ribcage and breathe 360 degrees.

The aim is to progress to inhaling for a count of five, exhaling for a count of five. You can work up to this, starting with breathing in and out to a count of three, four, then five.

The count of five will be used in the Hundred on page 176.

STARTING POSITION

Relaxation Position (page 37). This can also be done in upright positions. Place your hands on your lower ribcage, fingers reaching around the front, thumbs back around your sides.

ACTION

01/ Breathe fully and deeply into the back and sides of your ribcage for up to a count of five.

02/ Breathe out completely up to a count of five.

Repeat x 10.

Stop if you feel dizzy.

WATCHPOINTS

• Use appropriate core connection to control your alignment and movements.

• Keep your shoulders and neck relaxed.

• Focus on your ribs closing down and drawing together during the exhalation and the progressive expansion of the ribcage during the inhalation.

STARTING POSITION

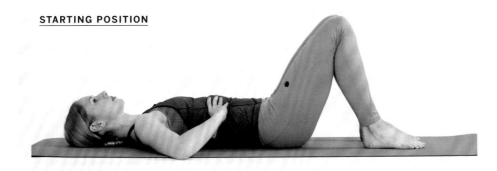

EXERCISE

Angel Wings Breathing

Try to make your exhalation longer than your inhalation to improve your vagal tone. Here we use the Double Floating Arms (page 75) movement of the arms to encourage better breathing.

STARTING POSITION

Relaxation Position (page 37), or any upright position. But first let's try it in Standing (page 50). Stand tall.

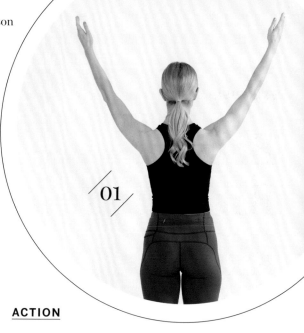

/01/

ACTION

01/ As you breathe in wide and deep, float both arms up in a wide arc as if you have Angel Wings. Lift to a count of four.

02/ Breathe out fully and completely as you lower your arms, following the same arc, for a count of six.

03/ In some positions, you could also combine it with a gentle upper back extension; see Standing Back Extension on page 116. Try to time the arm movements to coincide with your back extension.

STARTING POSITION

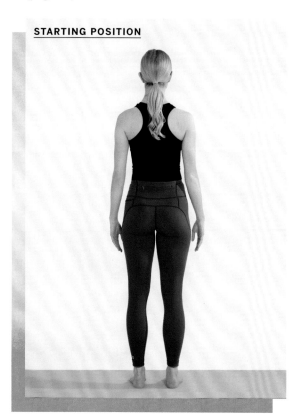

/03/

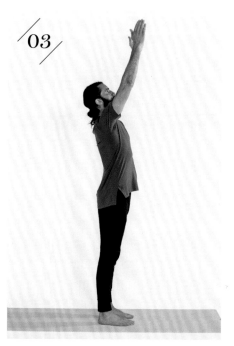

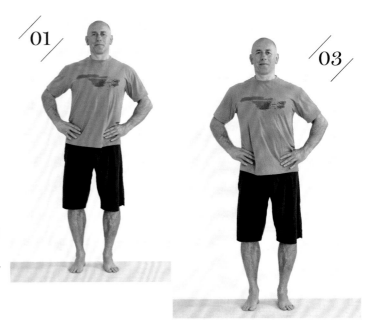

EXERCISE

Breathing Rib Shifts

Here we are asking you to direct your breath into one lung, or one side of the ribcage, and to open that side of the ribcage which will, hopefully, help you slide your ribcage across.

STARTING POSITION

Standing (page 50) or any upright position. Place your hands on the sides of your ribcage (or waist, if easier) with the thumbs around the back.

ACTION

01/ Breathe into your left lung/ribcage and use this opening of the ribs to help you shift your upper body to the left.

02/ Breathe out and shift your ribcage back to centre.

03/ Breathe into the right lung/ribcage and shift your ribcage to the right.

04/ Breathe out and shift it back to centre.

Repeat x 6 to each side, before returning to centre.

CHALLENGES & BENEFITS

• Challenges your ability to shift your upper body while keeping your pelvis stable.

• Promotes ribcage flexibility and better breathing.

WATCHPOINTS

• Use appropriate core connection to control your alignment and movements.

• Try to shift directly to the side and not twist or bend your spine in any other direction.

• Note that it is a small shift to the side.

• Keep both sides of your waist long and keep axial length throughout.

Advanced Rib Shifts

You can also do this exercise with your arms extended at shoulder height. Reach through your middle finger as you shift across.

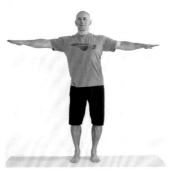

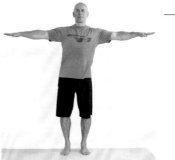

EXERCISE

Side Stretches

Designed to 'open' out your sides, this exercise can be done lying on your back or standing.

STARTING POSITION

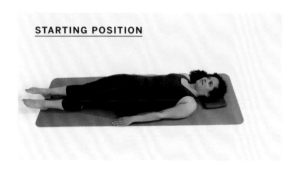

STARTING POSITION

Relaxation Position. With stability, stretch both legs out.

ACTION

01/ Breathe in to prepare.

02/ Breathe out and reach both arms up in a Ribcage Closure (page 73)

03/ Breathe in and cross your right leg over your left ankle.

04/ Breathe out and take your right hand across and clasp your left wrist. You are now in a long banana shape.

05/ Take advantage of the openness of your right side to take up to 6 deep breaths into the open ribcage.

06/ Then, slowly release your hand, uncross the legs and return to the Starting Position with control.

Repeat on the other side.

VARIATION:

You can increase the side stretch by moving the bottom of your ribs further away from your pelvis.

CHALLENGES & BENEFITS

• Challenges your awareness of good alignment.

• Opens out your sides, promoting flexibility of the ribcage and better breathing.

VARIATION

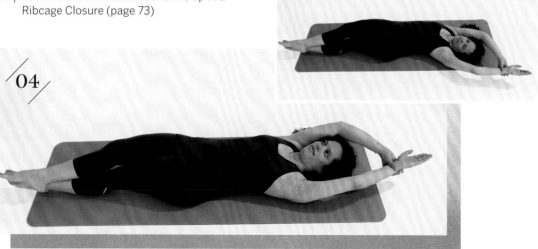

/04/

Standing Side Stretch

The vertical version.

STARTING POSITION

Stand tall on the floor. Cross your right foot over your left.

ACTION

01/ Breathe in to prepare and float both arms up, lightly clasp your right wrist with your left hand.

02/ Breathe out as you stretch up and over to the left, taking care not to shift your pelvis to the right as you do so.

03/ Breathe into the open side for 3 wide breaths, holding the stretch.

04/ Breathe out, closing the ribcage as you reach up and back to the centre.

05/ Breathe in as you lower your arms, then uncross your legs.

Repeat the sequence twice before repeating with the left foot crossed over the right foot. Then return with control to the Starting Position.

If you find this is too much of a challenge to your balance, you could try the stretch in a Split Stance position instead, or even simply Standing with your legs a bit wider than hip-width apart for added stability.

CHALLENGES & BENEFITS

As above, but with the added challenge to your balance and the resulting benefit of improving your balance.

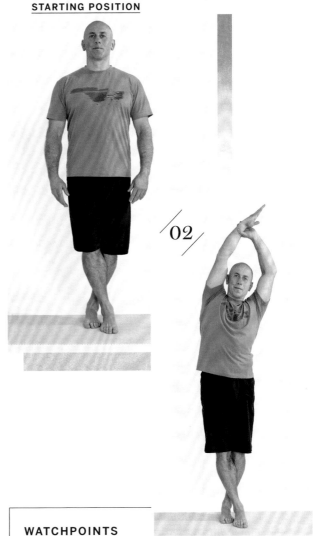

STARTING POSITION

/02/

WATCHPOINTS

- Use appropriate core connection to control your alignment and movements.

- Stay as centred as you can as you stretch.

- Really open out your sides; the ribs stretching away from the pelvis.

- Really breathe into the open side, then use the out breath to close the ribs down as you return to upright.

EXERCISE

Chest Expansion

We could not possibly have a chapter on respiratory health and leave out Chest Expansion – the name says it all! Once you have mastered the simple version, start combining it with other exercises.

STARTING POSITION

This exercise can be done in most upright positions, except seated on a mat as most arms are too long!

We will describe Standing. Stand tall, legs parallel and hip-width apart or connected in Pilates Stance (page 51). If using weights, hold a 2kg (4lb) weight in each hand and lengthen your arms down by your sides, palms facing backwards. If using a band, place it across the top of your thighs and hold it at a point where it gives you some, but not too much, resistance as you take your arms back.

ACTION

01/ Breathe in and, moving only from your shoulder joints, press your arms behind you, as far as is possible without disturbing the position of your spine.

02/ Still breathing in, turn your head to the left, then pass through centre and turn to the right.

03/ Breathe out as you return your head to the centre and lengthen your arms forwards, returning them slightly in front of the body.

Repeat up to x 8, alternating the side of the first head turn each time.

CHALLENGES & BENEFITS

• Challenges you to 'open' your chest without arching your back or flaring your ribs.

• Challenges you to co-ordinate your breath and movements.

• Challenges you to hold your breath without tension in the neck and shoulders.

• Mobilises your shoulders and neck.

• Expands the chest and ribcage; promoting better breathing.

WATCHPOINTS

• Use appropriate core connection to control your alignment and movements.

• Ensure that your upper back does not arch and your ribs do not flare as you press your arms behind you.

• As you turn your head, take care not to tip it back or forwards.

• Keep your hands and wrists in line with your forearms. Avoid rolling your fists away or towards you.

• Keep your chest and the front of your shoulders open, especially as you bring your arms forwards.

• Avoid locking out (hyper-extending) the elbows.

STARTING POSITION

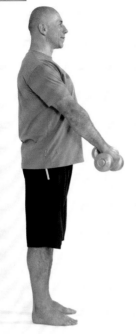

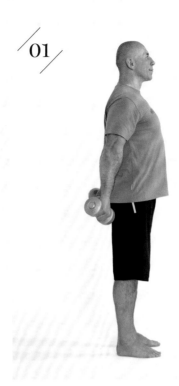

01

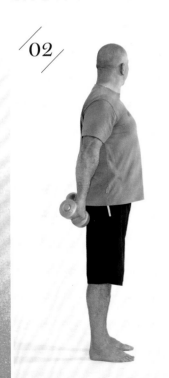

02

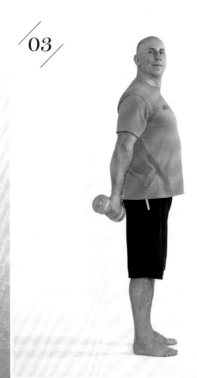

03

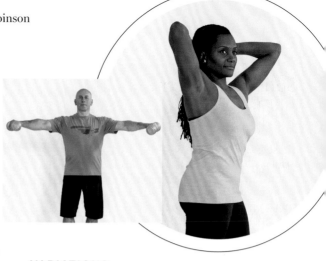

EXERCISE

Split Stance Twists

These are very functional movements – we stride and twist all the time. Here we are going to use rotation of the upper body to encourage an open ribcage and better breathing.

Split Stance Waist Twists

STARTING POSITION

Stand tall with your feet hip-width apart, then step forward with your right foot. Turn your back foot out so that the leg is turned out from your hip. (You can also try this with both legs in parallel.)

Your pelvis will rotate slightly back toward the back leg but try to keep it square. Keep your upper body facing forward ...for now. Fold your arms in front of your chest as for Waist Twists (page 86).

ACTION

01/ Breathe in wide to prepare.

02/ Breathe out as you rotate right, turning head, neck and ribs around. Pelvis as still as possible.

03/ Breathe in and turn to face centre.

04/ Breathe out and turn left.

05/ Breathe in as you turn back.

Repeat up to x 3 each way, then swap legs. Return to the Standing tall to finish.

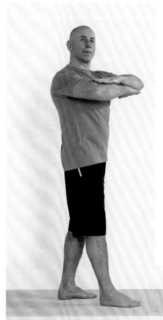

VARIATIONS

• As before but extend the arms to just below shoulder height. You could also hold weights.

• As before, but lightly clasp the hands behind your head.

• All the above, and you couldcome up onto your toes as you turn to mobilise and strengthen the ankles.

CHALLENGES & BENEFITS

• Challenge your balance, co-ordination and ability to twist, while lengthening the spine and pelvic stability.

• Works on the flexibility of your ribcage and your breathing.

• Mobilises your spine and hips.

• Works on your balance.

• Heel Raise version mobilises your ankles.

WATCHPOINTS

• Use appropriate core connection to control your alignment and movements.

• Lengthen up, up, up throughout as you move around your Centreline.

• Keep the weight even between both feet.

Split Stance Arm Circles with Twist

These feel so good, I have been getting up from writing at my computer every half hour to do them!

STARTING POSITION

As before, but have your arms relaxed by your sides.

ACTION

01/ Breathe in wide to your right ribcage as you circle your arm up and back, simultaneously turning head, neck and ribs to the right.

02/ Breathe out as your arm completes its circle back and down to the front, simultaneously turning your upper body back to face forwards.

03/ Repeat x 5 big circles, lengthening up as you spiral around.

Repeat the sequence but with the left foot forwards, right leg back, twisting this time to the left. Then step back to Standing tall to finish.

CHALLENGES & BENEFITS

In addition to those mentioned opposite:

• Mobilises the shoulders.

WATCHPOINTS

• Use appropriate core connection to control your alignment and movements.

• Allow the shoulders to move freely but do not over-reach with your arms.

• Try to time your arm circle so that you return to face forwards as the arm comes back by your side.

• Keep your weight even between both feet.

STARTING POSITION

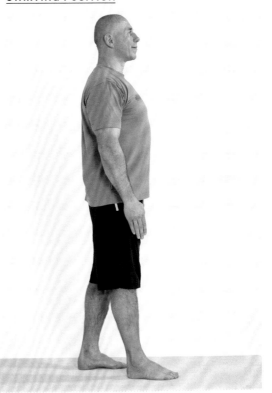

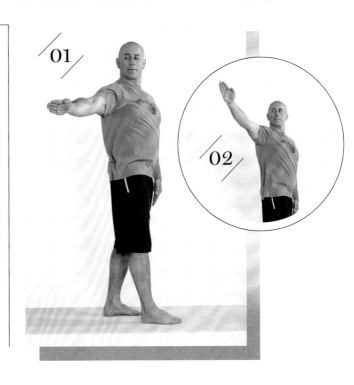

/ 01 /

/ 02 /

EXERCISE

Oblique Curl Ups

STARTING POSITION

Relaxation Position (page 37), With both hands clasped behind the head, elbows open but within your peripheral vision.

ACTION

01/ Breathe in to prepare.

02/ Breathe out and nod your head, then continue to sequentially curl up through the neck centrally. Once your head is lifted in line with your shoulders, rotate your trunk to the right in a diagonal line; left rib directed to right hip.

03/ Breathe in and curl up further.

04/ Breathe out and curl back down with control, reversing the diagonal line.

Repeat x 5 to each side. Alternate or repeat to the same side, if you prefer.

CHALLENGES & BENEFITS

As for Curl Ups on page 84, plus:

• Challenges your ability to curl up with length and precision, keeping your pelvis neutral.

• Works on rotation and therefore tones the waist.

• Mobilises the upper spine and ribcage, helping to improve breathing.

WATCHPOINTS

• Use appropriate core connection to control your alignment and movements.

• Your pelvis should be undisturbed.

• Keep your waist long on both sides.

• Visualise your lengthened Centreline as you rotate around it.

• Your head should remain heavy in the hands.

• Keep your shoulders relaxed, down and away from your ears.

STARTING POSITION

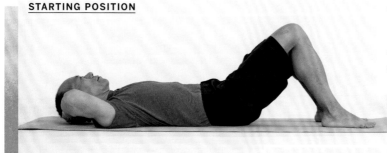

/02/

EXERCISE

Oblique Curls *with Rib Rolls*

A variation that seriously intensifies the work for your abdominals. You have been warned.

ACTION

Follow Action Points 1–2, then:

03/ Breathe in and twist your upper body to the left, rolling through your ribcage so that you end up with your right rib directed to your left hip.

04/ Breathe out and curl back down on the diagonal.

Repeat by curling up to the left this time and then rolling across to the right, before curling back down.

Alternate sides up to x 6.

CHALLENGES & BENEFITS

- Challenges your ability to rotate segmentally with length.

- Whittles down your waist.

- Mobilises your ribcage and upper spine and helps with your breathing.

WATCHPOINTS

As above, plus:

- Imagine rolling across the lower edge of your shoulder blades.

- Think ribs around, ribs around.

/03/

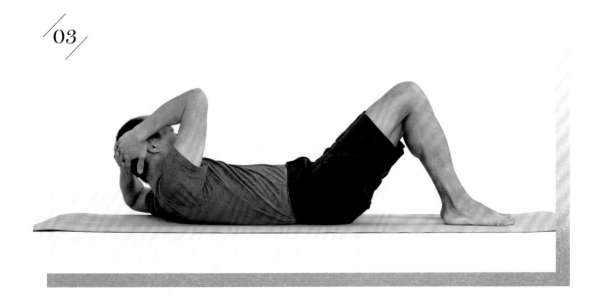

STARTING POSITION

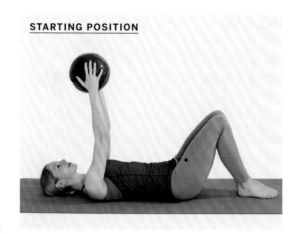

EXERCISE

Hip Rolls
with Rib Rolls

This exercise will mobilise your entire spine; this time, in rotation. If you have a medium ball or a Pilates Circle, it helps to hold it, but this is not essential. Note: The upper body rotation is not huge but nonetheless beneficial.

STARTING POSITION

Relaxation Position (page 37). Bring your legs together and connect your inner thighs. Reach your arms up over your shoulders, palms facing (or hold your ball/circle).

ACTION

01/ Breathe in to prepare.

02/ Breathe out, roll your pelvis to the right, simultaneously rolling your upper body to the left.

03/ Breathe in as you simultaneously return the pelvis, legs, ribs and arms to the Starting Position, initiating from your centre.

Repeat to the other side, then repeat the whole sequence up to x 5.

CHALLENGES & BENEFITS

• Challenges your ability to control your spinal rotation.

• Mobilises the entire axial length of the spine in rotation.

• Trims your waistline.

• Improves breathing by mobilising the upper spine and ribcage.

WATCHPOINTS

• Use appropriate core connection to control your alignment and movements.

• Roll your pelvis and legs directly to the side – avoid any detours.

• As you roll your ribcage, your head and neck come along with you.

• Keep both sides of your waist equally long.

/02/

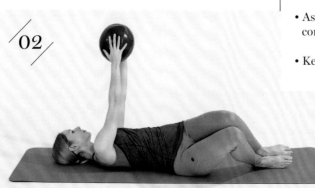

EXERCISE

Hip Rolls *with* Arm Circles

The multitasking here will be very useful when you do your mini workouts. Familiarise yourself with Arm Circles and Hip Rolls before combining them both.

Relaxation Position (page 37). Bring your legs together and connect your inner thighs. Lift your arms above your shoulders, palms facing away.

STARTING POSITION

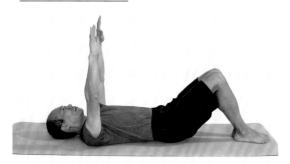

ACTION

01/ Breathe in to prepare.

02/ Breathe out as you hip roll to the left. Simultaneously, take both arms back in a Ribcage Closure (page 73) to about ear level.

03/ Breathe in and hold the position.

04/ Breathe out as you roll back to centre, simultaneously circling both arms back to the Starting Position.

Repeat x 5 to each side.

CHALLENGES & BENEFITS

• Challenges your ability to rotate the spine segmentally with control and length.

• Challenges your co-ordination.

• Mobilises the spine and shoulders.

• Tones your waistline.

WATCHPOINTS

• Use appropriate core connection to control your alignment and movements.

• Roll your pelvis and legs directly to the side – avoid any detours.

• Keep both sides of your waist equally long.

• As you roll, roll first through your hips, waist and lower ribs. Returning, roll through your lower ribs, waist and finally hips.

• Try to time your Hip Roll and Arm Circle so that your arms and hips arrive back in the Starting Position.

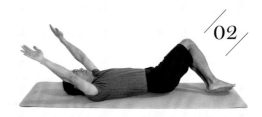

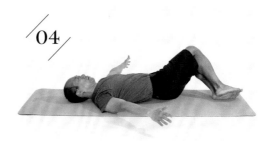

Threading the Needle

Another feel-good exercise with many benefits.

STARTING POSITION

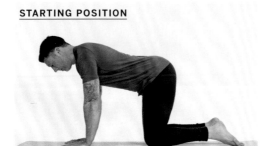

Four-point Kneeling (page 44).

ACTION

01/ Breathe in to prepare, transferring the weight to the left arm.

02/ Breathe out as you lift your right hand (keeping the back of the hand in contact with the mat), then, initiating with a turn of the head, rotate and reach left. Your left elbow will bend, as will your hips.

03/ Breathe in as you slide the right arm back, rotating the spine back to the centre. Replace the right hand on the mat.

Repeat x 5 to each side.

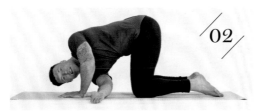

/02/

CHALLENGES & BENEFITS

• Challenges your ability to rotate segmentally, while keeping your pelvis still.

• Challenges the strength of your upper body.

• Mobilises the spine, shoulders and hips.

• Tones upper arms, shoulders and wrists.

• Encourages flexibility in the ribcage; improves breathing.

WATCHPOINTS

• The rotation of the spine is sequential. Initiate the movement with the head, neck then upper spine and return by initiating from the centre.

• Aim for axial length along and around your Centreline.

• Use appropriate core movements.

• Think long, long, long as you spiral round and back.

Moving on...

To challenge yourself further, try Threading the Needle with one leg stretched out along the mat in line with your hip. Tuck your toes under for extra stability. Stretch out the opposite leg to the hand that is lifted. This will work on your balance as well as your core stability.

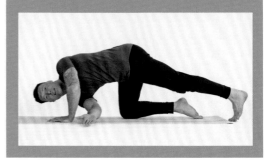

Threading the Needle Stretch

A fun variation on Threading the Needle, which really stretches out your waist.

STARTING POSITION

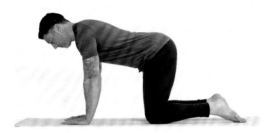

ACTION

01/ Breathe in to prepare, transferring the weight to the left arm.

02/ Breathe out as you slide your right hand forwards in line with your shoulder (keeping the palm in contact with the floor). Simultaneously twist your head, neck and ribcage left. Your left elbow will bend, as will your hips.

03/ Breathe in as you slide the right arm back, rotating the spine back to the centre. Replace the right hand on the mat.

Repeat x 5 to each side.

CHALLENGES & BENEFITS

As above, plus:

• Added stretch for the waist.

WATCHPOINTS

As above, plus:

• Try not to over-reach, it should be a gentle controlled stretch.

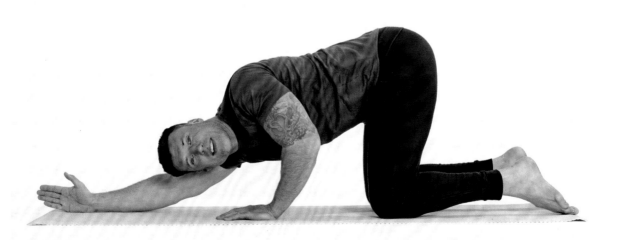

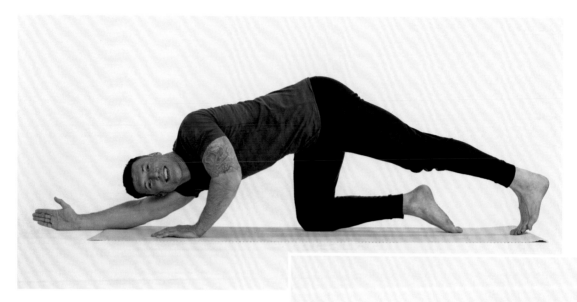

Advanced Threading the Needle Stretch

As before, you need to balance as you rotate. Follow the directions above, but this time with the opposite leg to stretching arm, lengthened away along the mat, tucking the toes under for added stability.

CHALLENGES & BENEFITS

As above, plus:

• Challenges your balance, stability and co-ordination.

WATCHPOINTS

As above, plus:

• Stay in control of the rotations; do not over-twist.

• Try to make the movements flow naturally.

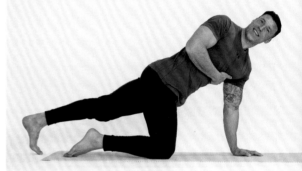

Advanced Threading the Needle Stretch and Twist

For additional challenge (should you require it) follow the directions 1-3 in Threading a Needle (with or without your leg stretched out) but instead of replacing your hand on the mat, wrap it around your ribs and twist the other way on one breath, before returning to the Starting Position.

EXERCISE

Opening Doors

This is a useful exercise, which is even better when combined with other exercises.

STARTING POSITION

Any upright position. Hold your arms out to the sides in line with your shoulders and bend your elbows at right angles, palms face forwards.

ACTION

01/ Breathe in to prepare.

02/ Breathe out and bring your arms forwards so that they are level in front of your shoulders. Allow your shoulder blades to move apart with control.

03/ Breathe in wide and full as you move the arms back to the Starting Position. Your shoulder blades will retract slightly.

Repeat up to x 6, making sure your shoulders do not creep up!

VARIATION:
One Arm Opening Doors

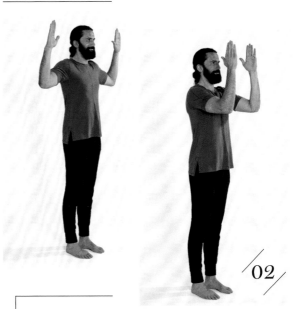

Move one arm at a time, alternating arms. As with all one-limb movements, you will have to focus on staying central and try to avoid rotating.

CHALLENGES & BENEFITS

• Challenges you to keep good postural alignment, especially shoulder alignment and stability.

• Works and stretches the muscles between and below your shoulder blades.

• Mobilises your shoulder joints.

• Opens the chest, which benefits your breathing.

WATCHPOINTS

• Use appropriate core connection to control your alignment and movements.

• Notice what happens to your shoulder blades as your arms move together – they move apart, your mid-back widens. Then they move back together as your arms return to the Starting Position. Try to make them glide smoothly in both directions.

• Maintain the distance between your ears and your shoulders as your arms move.

• Try to keep the elbows lifted and at right angles as you 'open' and 'close'.

• Keep your collarbones wide and open throughout.

EXERCISE

Opening Doors *with Flexion and Extension*

We racked our brains but this was the best title we could come up with. Thankfully, the exercise is more exciting than its title.

STARTING POSITION

As above, but have your knees slightly bent.

ACTION

01/ Breathe in to prepare.

02/ Breathe out and, as you bring your arms forwards, sequentially curl your spine, head, neck and upper spine into a standing Curl Up.

03/ Breathe in and, as you move the arms back to the Starting Position, sequentially from the bottom up, extend your upper spine until you are in a gentle Standing Back Bend (page 92).

Repeat up to x 6, before lengthening back sequentially to upright.

STARTING POSITION

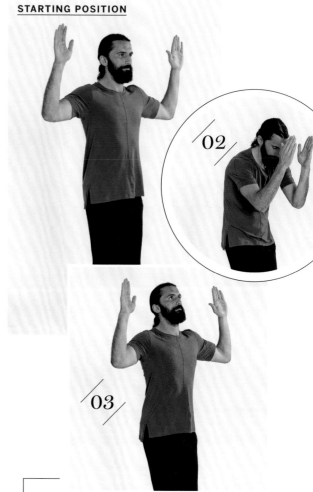

CHALLENGES & BENEFITS

As above, plus:

• Challenges you to control the flexion and extension of your upper spine with axial length.

• Mobilises your upper spine; promoting better breathing.

WATCHPOINTS

As above, plus:

• Move through your Centreline, taking care not to over-flex or over-extend your spine.

• Your pelvis stays still; your weight central.

EXERCISE

Mermaid

Always popular, this stretches and works the waist. You can vary the Starting Position as not everyone finds the traditional version comfortable.

STARTING POSITION

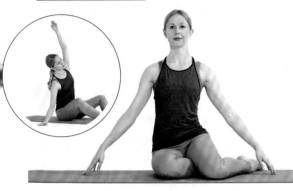

There are options here. If you have back, knee or hip problems, you may prefer to sit in Long Frog (page 42).

For the traditional version, kneel on the mat, sitting back onto your heels. Then move your pelvis off the heels to the right and onto the mat. If necessary, open your knees slightly so your legs are comfortable.

Try to keep your pelvis as level as possible. Lengthen and lift your spine from a strong centre.

ACTION

01/ Breathe in as you float your left arm up.

02/ Breathe out as you reach up and over to the right. Your right arm will slide further along the mat.

03/ Breathe into your open side.

04/ Breathe out as you straighten the right arm and return to upright. Lower your left arm and return it to the mat.

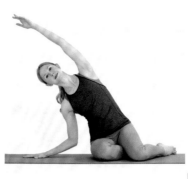
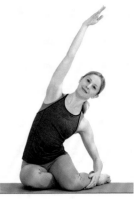

05/ Repeat to the other side, though note the stretch is minimal to this side.

Repeat x 3 stretches to each side, then swap your pelvis and legs across to the other side and repeat the sequence.

CHALLENGES & BENEFITS

• Challenges you to control your side flexion.

• Mobilises your spine and ribcage.

• Encourages lateral breathing.

• Stretches and works the waist.

• The traditional Starting Position mobilises your hips and knees.

WATCHPOINTS

• Use appropriate core connection to control your alignment and movements.

• When you reach to the side, your spine and arm should move as one.

• When side bending, initiate the movement with your head, followed sequentially by your neck and upper spine. As you return, initiate the movement from your centre.

• Try to move in one plane only and not curve forwards or arch back.

• Keep your head and neck in line with the rest of your spine.

EXERCISE

Mermaid
with Rib Rolls

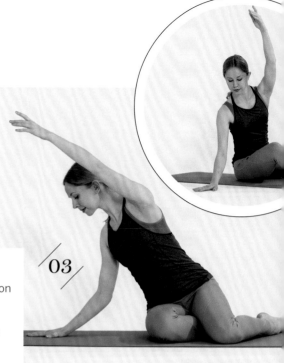

A challenging version based on an exercise we do on the studio Wunda Chair. This version increases the mobilisation of the upper and mid-spine and the ribcage.

Note: You will not rotate 'back and up' very far – do not force the movement.

Double note: You are only stretching one way at a time here.

STARTING POSITION

As above, this can be done with the legs to one side or in Long Frog.

ACTION

Follow Action Points 1–2 above, then:

03/ As you breathe in, rotate your upper body downwards to the right. One 'lung' moves forwards, one backwards. Think Rib Rolls (page 109). Your raised arm only moves reactively.

04/ Breathe out as you rotate back to face forwards again.

05/ Breathe in to rotate up and back to the left; again one 'lung' moves forwards, one back.

06/ Breathe out as you rotate to face forwards.

07/ Breathe out as you return to upright.

Repeat x 3 to this side before lowering the arm. Swap your pelvis and legs and repeat on the other side.

CHALLENGES & BENEFITS

• Challenges your ability to side flex and rotate the spine segmentally with length.

• Mobilises spine, ribs and hips.

WATCHPOINTS

• Use appropriate core connection to control your alignment and movements

• Your head moves in sync and in line with your spine.

• As you side bend and rotate, try to keep your pelvis centred.

• Spiral up, up, up as you rotate; axial length along and around your Centreline.

EXERCISE

The Dart

This really ought to be placed in The New Fundamentals section, but we are going to work on a lot of variations, so it was easier to place it here. Read through the directions carefully. We have simplified the leg position to be the same for each variation.

STARTING POSITION

Prone (page 48). Place a folded towel or flat cushion underneath the forehead. Your arms are lengthened down your sides, resting on the mat, palms facing up. Your legs are lengthened, turned out from the hips, and hip- or shoulder-width apart.

ACTION

01/ Breathe in to prepare.

02/ Breathe out as you lift first your head, then neck and upper spine, one vertebra at a time. At the same time, lengthen your arms away and lift them slightly, turning your palms to face the body.

03/ Breathe in and maintain this lengthened position.

04/ Breathe out as you sequentially return to the mat, while simultaneously turning your arms back to the Starting Position.

Repeat up to x 8.

CHALLENGES & BENEFITS

• Challenges you to extend your spine sequentially, with pelvic stability.

• Works your back and gluteal muscles.

• Mobilises your upper spine, hips and shoulders.

• Improves your postural endurance, helping you breathe better.

WATCHPOINTS

• Use appropriate core connection to control your alignment and movements.

• Take care not to tip your head back too far – your gaze remains down throughout.

• Ensure the right order of events: first the head lifts, then the neck and when they are in line with the upper spine, then the upper spine extends. Your ribs stay connected down into your waist.

• Do not be tempted to lift the legs; they stay grounded.

STARTING POSITION

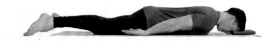

/02/

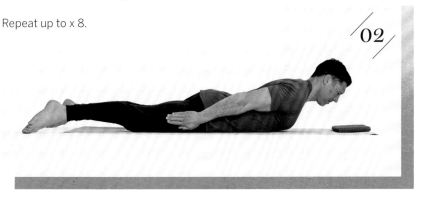

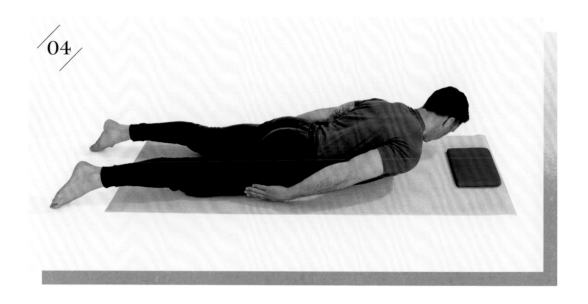

Dart into Side Bend

When you are planning a mini workout, it is incredibly useful to be able to combine back extension with side flexion so you tick two boxes with one exercise.

STARTING POSITION

As for Dart.

ACTION

Follow Action points 1–3 above, then:

04/ Breathe out and, leading with your head, neck and upper back, side bend to the left, keeping your pelvis central and hovering your breastbone just off the mat in one plane.

05/ Breathe in as you lengthen up and return to the centre.

Repeat x 2 to each side before lowering back down to the Starting Position with control.

CHALLENGES & BENEFITS

As for Dart, plus:

- Challenges your ability to side bend into extension in one plane of movement.

- Mobilises the upper spine into side flexion as well as into extension.

- Opens the side of your ribcage and waist, thus promoting more flexibility and better breathing.

- Works and stretches your waist.

WATCHPOINTS

- Use appropriate core connection to control your alignment and movements.

- Return to your Centreline before you bend to the other side.

- Keep both feet on the ground throughout.

- If it is more comfortable, place a flat folded towel under your abdomen.

Dart with Salute

We have upped the challenge here by lifting the arm. This increases the load considerably, which increases the work for your back muscles.

STARTING POSITION

As above.

ACTION

Follow Action points 1–2 above, then:

03/ Breathe in and float one arm out to the side and above you. Keep the arm off the ground at shoulder level as it moves. Bring the back of your hand to salute your forehead.

04/ Breathe out as you straighten your arm and bring it back down by your side. Maintain your back extension.

Repeat x 2, alternating arms, before returning slowly to the Starting Position, sequentially and with control.

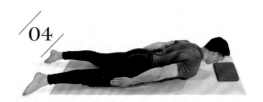

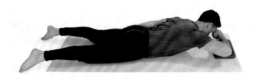

Dart with Salute into Side Bend

Not a stunning name for an exercise, but at least you know what you are doing. Follow the directions opposite, but simply side bend with your hand resting on your forehead in a salute, rather than down by your side.

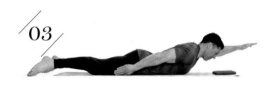

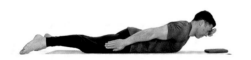

CHALLENGES & BENEFITS

• Challenges you to extend your spine sequentially, with stability and then maintain the extension.

• Works your back, gluteal and shoulder muscles.

• Mobilises your upper spine, shoulders and elbows.

WATCHPOINTS

• Use appropriate core connection to control your alignment and movements.

• There is a lot going on in these versions. Stay in control of each component part.

• Your arms should float, moving freely just above the floor.

• Maintain the distance between your ears and shoulders.

• Both sides of your waist lengthen as you side bend.

• Your legs stay grounded.

Exercises for a *Healthy Immune System*

In this chapter we will be looking at exercises to keep your immune system healthy. It is movement that stimulates the lymphatic system and, thus, the immune system. We are looking, in particular, to mobilise those joints that have a lot of lymph nodes nearby.

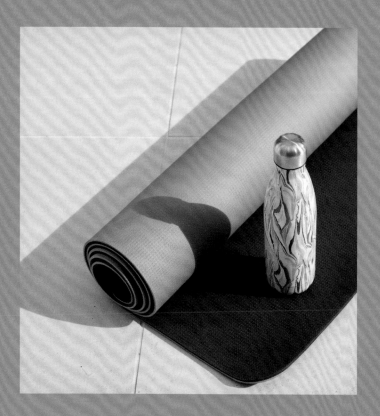

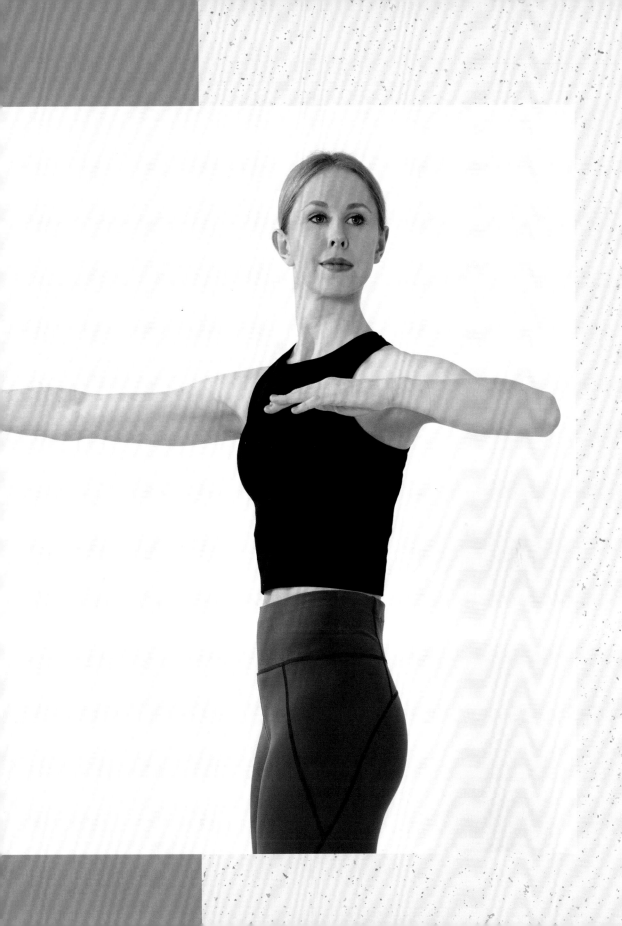

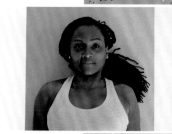

EXERCISE

Rainbow Necks

There are a lot of lymph nodes around the neck and collarbones, so we want to gently mobilise the area. We dedicate this exercise to our wonderful UK NHS staff and all the medical personnel around the world who worked so bravely and tirelessly through the pandemic.

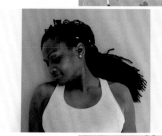

STARTING POSITION

Relaxation Position (page 37), arms resting by your sides. Have a flat cushion or folded towel under your head if needed, but it should not be tipping your head forwards; see page 55 for good neck alignment. This exercise can also be done in a Seated position (page 42), but we recommend practising it first with your head supported by the floor.

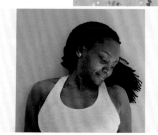

ACTION

Breathe slowly and deeply throughout, following your own timing.

01/ With control, roll your head and neck directly to one side.

02/ Tilt your chin down towards your armpit, as if you intend to sniff it – do not lift your head. This is the start of your rainbow.

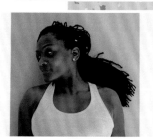

03/ Then, with your head, follow the arc of the rainbow up across to the other side. You should end up in a mirror position to position 2.

04/ Slowly trace your rainbow back and forth.

Repeat up to x 8. Finish in the centre with a gentle Chin Tuck (page 40), nodding the head forwards, drawing the chin down and lengthening the back of your neck. Return to the Starting Position.

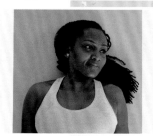

WATCHPOINTS

CHALLENGES & BENEFITS

• Challenges your ability to roll smoothly and segmentally through your neck vertebra.

• Mobilises the neck, thus stimulating lymph flow.

• Aim for a smooth, even, synchronised arc.

• Do not push or strain; allow the gentle movement to mobilise your neck.

• Stay wide and open across your collarbones.

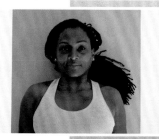

EXERCISE

Nose Spirals

I love this one. I find it especially helpful if I feel a tension headache coming on.

STARTING POSITION

Relaxation Position (page 37), arms lengthened down by your sides. You can open or close your eyes. You could also do this exercise in an upright position, like Seated (page 42–3) or High Kneeling (page 46).

ACTION

Breathe normally throughout.

01/ Imagine the centre of a circle hovering just above your nose. Slowly, with control, start to circle your head, making each circle slightly larger than the last, as you spiral outwards.

02/ Stop when you have reached your outer circle, then start to spiral back, in ever decreasing circles, to the Starting Position.

03/ Finish the exercise with a gentle Chin Tuck (page 40), nodding the head forwards, drawing the chin down and lengthening the back of your neck. Return to the Starting Position.

Repeat up to x 6 clockwise and anticlockwise.

CHALLENGES & BENEFITS

- Challenges you to control the smooth movement of your neck.

- Mobilises the neck and helps free tension in the area.

- Encourages lymph flow.

WATCHPOINTS

- Try not to disturb the natural, neutral curves of your upper and lower back.

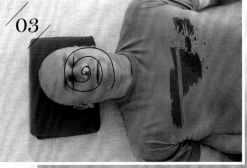

03

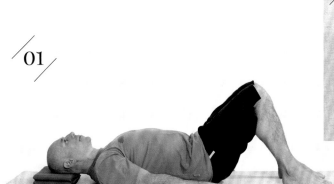

01

EXERCISE

Spine Twirls

Another variation on our popular Spine Curls (page 78). This adds rotation into the mix. Although you are rotating the pelvis, be aware of your Centreline and rotate around it.

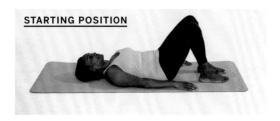

STARTING POSITION

Relaxation Position (page 37), arms lengthened down by the side of your body.

CHALLENGES & BENEFITS

As above, plus:

• A greater challenge to your spinal and pelvic stability.

• Challenges your awareness of your Centreline.

• Targets your hips more than standard Spine Curls; mobilising them more.

• Your gluteal muscles need to work much harder in this version, because you stay up longer.

WATCHPOINTS

• Use appropriate core connection to control your alignment and movements.

• Try to roll the same amount to each side.

• Avoid swaying across to one side; roll directly around your Centreline.

ACTION

01/ Breathe in to prepare.

02/ Breathe out as you curl your tailbone under and roll your spine up segmentally to the tips of the shoulder blades.

03/ Breathe in and hold this position.

04/ Breathe out and tilt your pelvis to one side, dipping down but without losing height or shortening your waist.

05/ Breathe in and tilt back to centre.

06/ Breathe out and tilt the other way.

07/ Breathe in, back to centre.

08/ Breathe out and roll down just a few vertebrae.

09/ Repeat tilting to each side and then rolling down a segment x 3.

10/ Then, when centred, roll back down into neutral.

Repeat up to x 5.

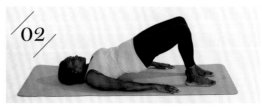

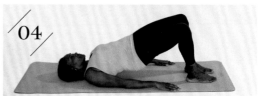

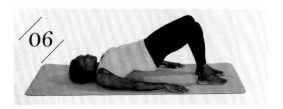

EXERCISE

Windows

Windows is a useful exercise for mobilising your shoulders. It rotates your shoulder joint; a useful exercise for mobilising your shoulders and stimulating surrounding lymph nodes.

STARTING POSITION

Relaxation Position (page 37). Raise both arms above the chest, wrists directly above the shoulders, palms facing forwards.

ACTION

01/ Breathe in to prepare.

02/ Breathe out as you bend both elbows towards the mat, keeping your elbows in line with your shoulders.

03/ Breathe in as you rotate your arms to lower the forearms back towards the floor.

04/ Breathe out as you straighten your arms, reaching them behind you.

Repeat up to x 5.

STARTING POSITION

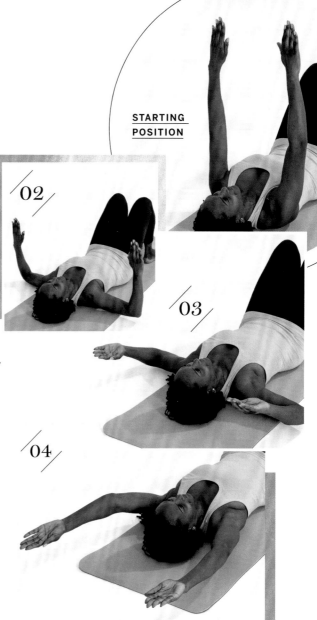

CHALLENGES & BENEFITS

• Challenges your ability to isolate the movement at the shoulder without disturbing the spine.

• Encourages stability and mobility of the shoulder joints; strengthening and mobilising the muscles around the shoulders.

• Mobilises your elbows.

• Encourages lymph flow.

WATCHPOINTS

• Use appropriate core connection to control your alignment and movements.

• At no point should your arms (including elbows) touch the floor.

• Your upper spine remains undisturbed, your ribs connected. Think Ribcage Closure (page 73).

Standing Windows into Opening Doors

Opening Doors, Windows... if nothing else, you will be well ventilated! A great combination exercise that works best in an upright position. The combination is more challenging than the original exercises.

STARTING POSITION

Stand tall (or in any upright position). Hold your arms out in front of your shoulders at just below shoulder height, palms facing down.

CHALLENGES & BENEFITS

As for Windows (page 127) and Opening Doors (page 115), plus:

• Challenges your awareness of where your arms are in space.

• Challenges your ability to stay in control of your postural alignment.

• Mobilises the shoulders and elbows and builds endurance into your shoulders and upper body.

• Improves breathing and lymph flow.

WATCHPOINTS

• Use appropriate core connection to control your alignment and movements.

• Stay aware of your postural alignment as your arms move.

• Think collarbones wide and open throughout, neck long.

• Try not to allow your shoulders to roll forwards as you rotate the upper arms.

• Keep checking your elbows have not dropped too far below your shoulders.

ACTION

01/ Breathe in to prepare.

02/ Breathe out and draw both arms back, bending your elbows so that your upper arms are in line with your shoulders.

03/ Breathe in and rotate your upper arms, keeping the elbows still in space. This will bring you into the Opening Doors Starting Position.

04/ Breathe out and bring your arms forwards to shoulder-width apart.

05/ Breathe in and open the arms back to the side.

06/ Breathe out and rotate the upper arms again, so that your palms face down.

07/ Breathe in and extend both arms forwards to the Starting Position.

Repeat up to x 5.

STARTING POSITION

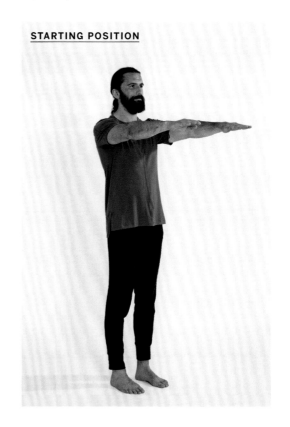

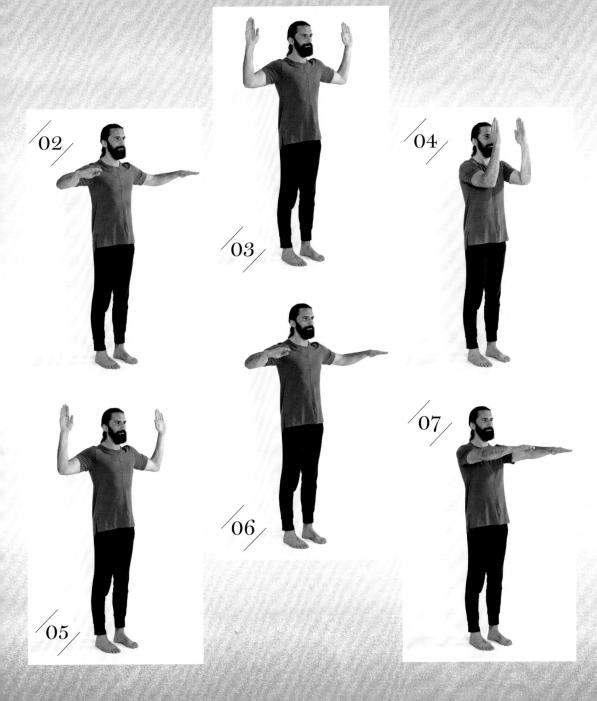

EXERCISE

Rolling Chalk Circles

Just looking at the photos of this exercise should make you feel better. The sheer joy of rolling around the floor. Simple pleasures.

STARTING POSITION

Relaxation Position (page 37) but with a substantial cushion under your head (a bed pillow is perfect). Feet together.

ACTION

01/ Breathe in and roll your knees across to the right. Simultaneously start to move your left hand across your hips to start the circle.

02/ Breathe out as you roll onto your right side, knees still together. Your left arm will continue its circle upwards.

03/ Breathe in as you reach up and overhead.

04/ Breathe out when you have to start rolling your body and knees back to the centre position. Your arm continues its circle down and around to the Starting Position.

05/ Breathe in as your knees roll left; your right arm starting to circle over your hip.

06/ Breathe out as you roll onto your left side, knees still together; your right arm will continue its circle.

07/ Breathe in as you reach up and overhead.

08/ Breathe out when you have to start rolling back to the centre position. Your arm continues its circle down and around to the Starting Position.

Repeat as many times as you like!

CHALLENGES & BENEFITS

• Challenges you to Roll with Control

• Promotes sequential rotation of the spine and shoulder mobility.

• Stimulates lymph flow in neck, chest, armpits and trunk.

If you find the breathing pattern difficult, just breathe normally.

WATCHPOINTS

• Use appropriate core connection to control your alignment and movements

• Enjoy the movements, let it flow with control, and take care not to over-reach your arm or over-arch your back.

STARTING POSITION

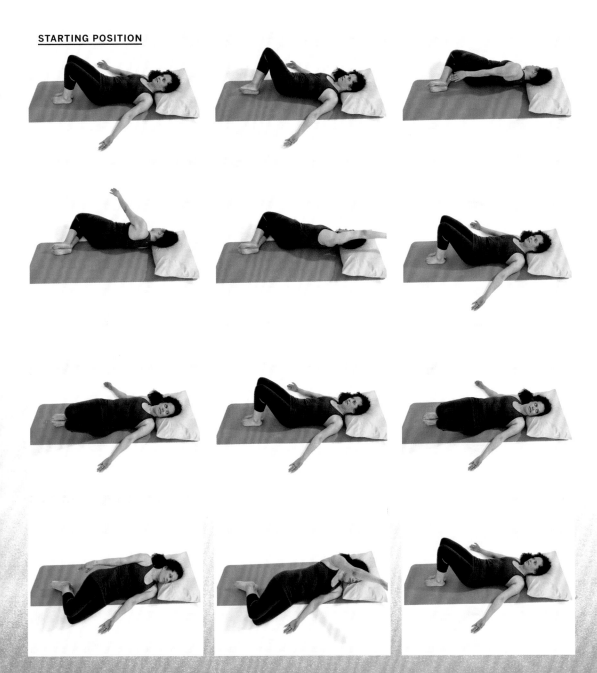

EXERCISE

Walking *on the* Spot

You can do this exercise Standing or Seated on a Chair (see opposite). Your leg alignment is crucial. Feet must be hip-width apart, parallel. Spine lengthened. Head balanced over ribcage, over pelvis. Visualise your Centreline.

CHALLENGES & BENEFITS

• Challenges your postural alignment head to toe.

• Mobilises hips, knees and ankles.

• Works your feet.

• Stimulates lower limb circulation and thus lymph flow.

STARTING POSITION

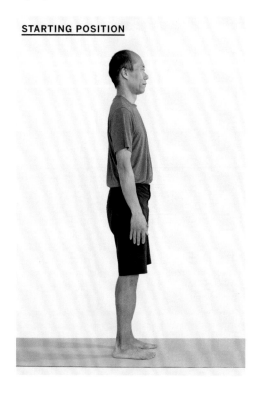

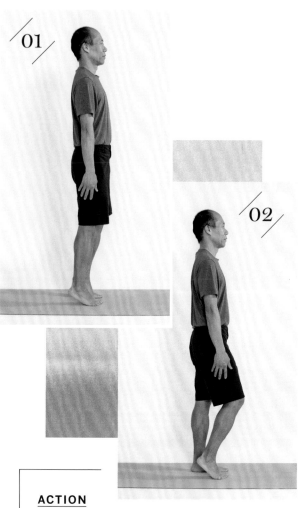

ACTION

Breathing normally throughout both versions.

Standing

01/ Come up onto your toes, lifting both heels.

02/ Bend one knee, sending it directly forwards, lowering the other heel back onto the floor.

03/ Immediately, transfer your weight, swapping legs.

04/ Allow your arms to relax down by your sides.

Repeat walking on the spot until you feel suitably warmed up.

Seated Walking on the Spot

Two options here: you can simply alternate heel lifts in a similar action to the Standing version or you can opt for the heel/toe version.

VERSION 2: TOE/HEEL

01/ Simultaneously lift the heel of one foot and the toes of the other foot. Swap.

02/ Repeat either version until your legs feel suitably warmed up.

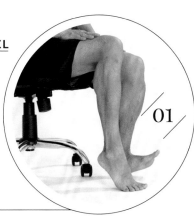

STARTING POSITION

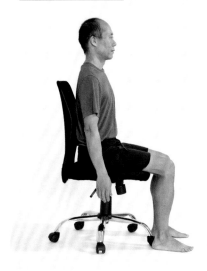

Shift to the front of the chair to give your knees and hips room. Weight even on both sitting bones. Spine lengthened in neutral.

WATCHPOINTS

- Use appropriate core connection to control your alignment and movements.

- It is very important to roll through the feet with all the versions: heel, ball, toe, then reverse.

- Your ankles and knees must not roll in or out.

- Maintain good alignment of the rest of your body too. Keep both sides of your waist equally long throughout.

- If standing, do not sink into one hip when the heel drops; think up, up, up through your Centreline.

VERSION 1: WALKING

01/ Lift one heel, directing the front of your ankle forwards over your second toe and rolling through your foot to come onto the ball of the foot.

02/ As you replace the heel, simultaneously lift the opposite heel.

Sounds more complicated than it is...

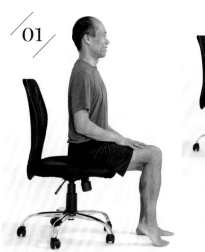

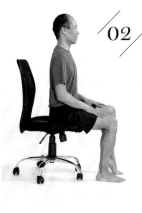

EXERCISE

Standing Speedy Warm-up

By speedy we do not mean rushed, but this fun exercise targets multiple joints and is a great way to warm up. It may conjure up memories of Keep Fit classes. Remember to apply your Pilates principles, you can prepare your body for the upcoming workout in a very short time! You will be marching on the spot but think of it as a Standing Knee Fold so that you stay in control of your pelvis and spine.

STARTING POSITION

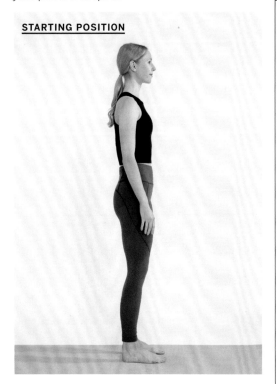

Stand tall, feet hip-width apart.

ACTION

Breathe normally throughout.

01/ Transferring your weight onto your right leg, fold your left knee up.

02/ Replace the foot. Repeat with the other leg. This sets up a marching action...

03/ March on the spot for a minute or so, then add an arm action and a twist.

04/ As you fold your right knee up, swing your left arm across to tap the outside of your right thigh – allow your trunk to rotate right as you do this.

05/ Lengthen up as you return to face the front. As the foot returns to the floor, the arm swings back and you repeat to the other side.

Repeat up to x 10 alternating sides, arms and legs.

CHALLENGES & BENEFITS

• Challenges you to move mindfully.

• Mobilises your hips, ankles, knees, shoulders and spine. Mobilises the ribcage; encouraging efficient breathing.

• Gets lymph flowing.

WATCHPOINTS

• Use appropriate core connection to control your alignment and movements.

• Good leg alignment is paramount.

• Lengthen up through your Centreline throughout. Keep both sides of your waist lifted and lengthened.

• Try to roll through the foot as you lift it as for Walking on the Spot (page 132), directing the front of your ankle over your second toe.

• Fold the knees up as high as you can without disturbing the neutral position of your pelvis.

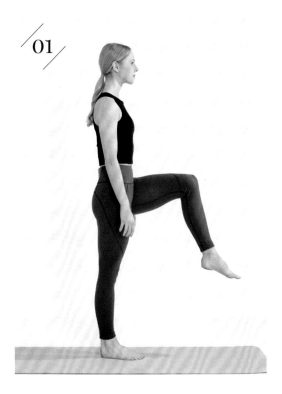

01

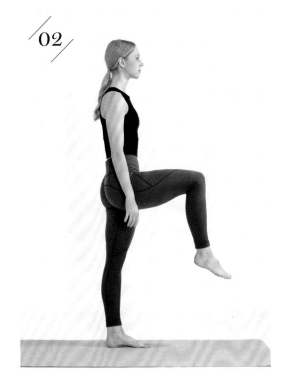

02

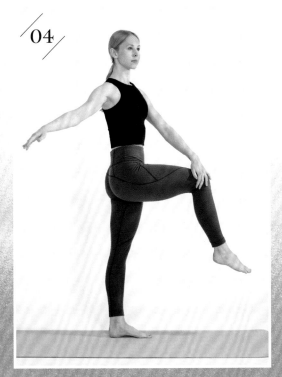

04

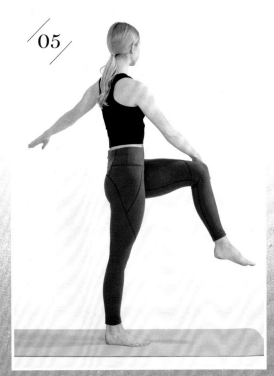

05

STARTING POSITION

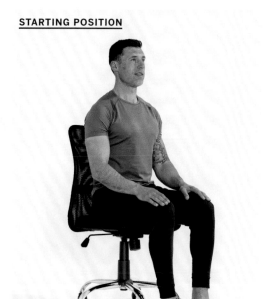

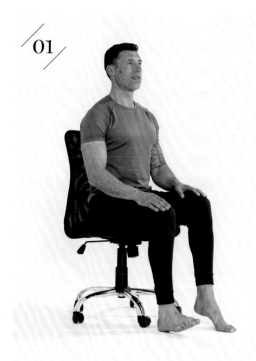

/01/

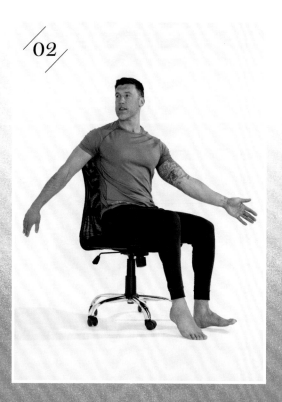

/02/

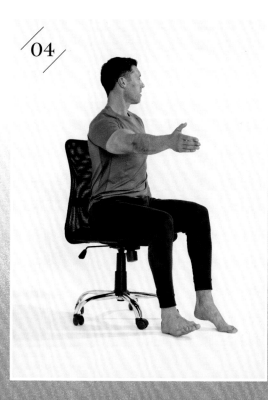

/04/

EXERCISE

Seated Speedy Warm-up

A fun variation for when you cannot stand up! You can use either food action from page 133. Here we've show you Version 2.

STARTING POSITION

Sit tall towards the front of a sturdy chair, preferably one without arms. (See below for alternative version if your chair has arms). Feet hip-width apart. Arms relaxed.

ACTION

Breathe normally throughout again...

01/ Lift alternate toes/heels so that you are 'walking 'on the spot. Take care that you are rolling through the foot, directing the front of your ankles forward, not rolling in or out.

Once you have established your walking pattern and your lower legs feel warmed up, add an arm action and twist...

02/ As your right heel/left toes lift, turn your head, neck, and upper spine to the right, allowing your right arm to swing back, your left arm forward.

03/ Return to face front as your heel/toes lower.

04/ Immediately, lift your left heel/right toes, rotating your trunk to the left, your right arm swings forward, left arm back.

05/ Return to face front again as your heel/toes lower again.

Repeat for a few minutes until you can feel the benefits.

CHAIR WITH ARMS:

Rest your hands lightly on your thighs, then instead of swinging your arms, slide them back and forth on top of your legs.

CHALLENGES & BENEFITS

- Challenges your brain with lefts/rights!

WATCHPOINTS

- Use appropriate core connection to control your alignment and movements.

- Spiral up, up, up as you rotate around your Centreline.

- Keep your weight even on both sitting bones.

- Keep your pelvis still and stable.

- Try to rotate sequentially each time; do not twist the neck too far.

- If you lose the walking pattern, getting confused with lefts and rights (as I often do); just pause and reset.

EXERCISE

The Wave

This flowing exercise flexes the spine from both ends, mobilising spine and hips. It is advisable to be familiar with both Curl Ups (page 84) and Spine Curls (page 78). Timing is everything. The goal is to arrive in the finished Spine Curl position just as your head touches down, and the finished Curl Up position, as your tailbone lands.

STARTING POSITION

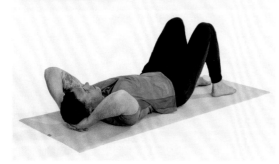

Relaxation Position (page 37). Lightly clasp your hands behind your head, ensuring that you do not arch your upper back as you do so. Have your elbows open and positioned just in front of your ears and within your peripheral vision.

ACTION

01/ Breathe in to prepare.

02/ Breathe out as you lengthen the back of your neck, nod your head and sequentially curl your upper body from your mat. Keep your lower ribcage in contact with the mat.

03/ Breathe into the back of the ribcage to maintain the position.

04/ Breathe out and, as you start to roll your upper body back down, simultaneously roll your tailbone under and sequentially curl up from the bottom end – tailbone to shoulder blades. (See note on timing above.)

03/ Breathe in and hold the Spine Curl.

04/ Breathe out and, as you start to roll the spine back down bone by bone, simultaneously, nod your head and start to Curl Up from the top end.

Repeat this spinal 'wave' up to x 8 before settling back down.

CHALLENGES & BENEFITS

As for Curl Ups and Spine Curls, plus:

• Challenges your awareness of where your spine starts and finishes.

• Challenges your co-ordination and timing.

• Mobilises spine and hips.

• Tones your abdominals and gluteal muscles.

WATCHPOINTS

As for Curl Ups and Spine Curls.

/02/

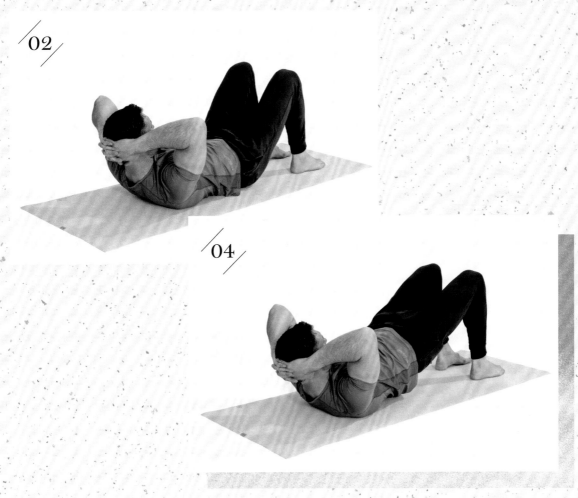

/04/

/05/

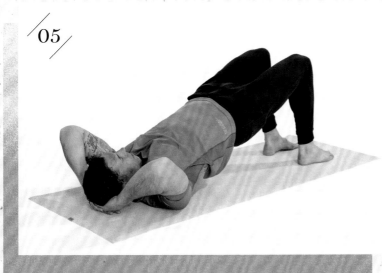

EXERCISE

Curl Ups with Variations

I always think a Curl Up is like a basic dish, say an omelette, which is simple yet hard to perfect, but once you have, you can then add lots of extra ingredients to liven it up.

Curl Ups with Knee Fold and Extension

As a teacher, I am always looking for ways to 'jazz up' Curl Ups. This version prepares you for Single Leg Stretch (page 171).

Relaxation Position (page 37), hands clasped lightly behind your head.

ACTION

01/ Breathe in to prepare.

02/ Breathe out as you nod your head and sequentially

03/ Breathe in and fold one knee up, without disturbing the pelvis.

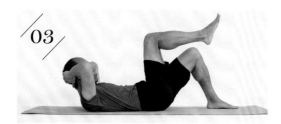

04/ Breathe out as you extend that leg to about 45 degrees (see Watchpoints), keeping it in line with your hip.

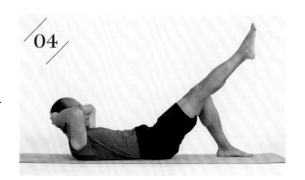

05/ Breathe in and bend the knee in again.

06/ Breathe out and replace the foot on the floor.

07/ Breathe in as you curl back down sequentially, with control, to the mat.

08/ Repeat the Curl Up, moving the other leg.

Repeat up to x 4 with each leg.

CHALLENGES & BENEFITS

As for Curl Ups (page 84) and Knee Folds (page 64), plus:

- Challenges your proprioception (awareness of where your joints are in space).

- Greater challenge to your core stability as the straightened leg adds extra load.

- Mobilises your hips and knees, and works your thigh muscles.

WATCHPOINTS

- Use appropriate core connection to control your alignment and movements.

- Do not lose the height of your Curl Up as your legs move.

- Breathe into the back of the ribcage to help you stay curled up.

- Fold the knee in and extend the leg as far as you can without disturbing the pelvis.

Curl Ups with Double Knee Openings

This exercise needs extra vigilance as it would be all too easy to lose a neutral pelvis as the knees open and return. Stay in control!

STARTING POSITION.

As above.

ACTION

Follow directions 1–2 above.

03/ Breathe in and open both knees to the side as for Knee Openings (page 63). Do not open them so far that you disturb your pelvis and spine.

04/ Breathe out and bring your knees back to parallel.

05/ Breathe in and curl back down.

Repeat up to x 6

CHALLENGES & BENEFITS

As for Curls Ups and Knee Openings, plus:

• Challenges your ability to maintain neutral pelvis and stay in control of your lumbar spine.

WATCHPOINTS

• Use appropriate core connection to control your alignment and movements.

• Roll your feet onto their outer borders as you open the knees.

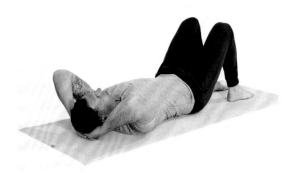

/03/

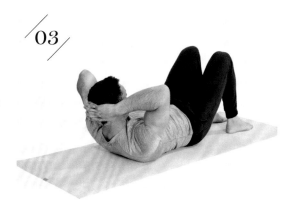

/04/

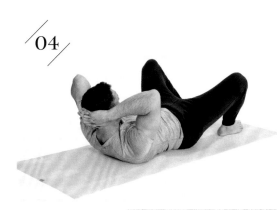

Moving on...

You could stay in the Curl Up position as you repeat a few Double Knee Openings.

EXERCISE

Rocking Cat

A wonderful exercise. Do not be put off by the long list of ingredients, oops directions, the exercise flows naturally. If necessary, refresh your memory of Cat (page 80).

STARTING POSITION

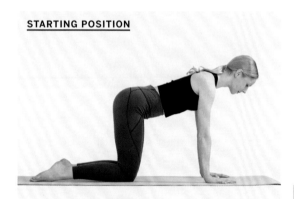

Four-point Kneeling (page 44).

ACTION

01/ Breathe in and lengthen your spine.

02/ Breathe out as you roll your pelvis underneath you and sequentially round the spine into an elongated C-Curve.

03/ Breathe in as you move your body, back towards your heels, folding at the hips and maintaining your C-Curve shape.

04/ Breathe out and move forwards again, still in a C-Curve.

05/ Breathe in as you start to unravel the spine, sending the tailbone away from the crown of your head, returning to neutral.

06/ Breathe out and gently start to extend your upper spine, lengthening through first your head, then neck and shining your breastbone forwards collarbones wide and open, into reverse C-Curve.

07/ Breathe in and, folding at the hips again, move your spine and pelvis backwards to your heels, keeping as much of the spinal extension as you can (see below).

08/ Breathe out and move forward again, maintaining the reverse C-Curve.

09/ Breathe in and lengthen back into neutral.

Repeat up to x 6.

VARIATION:

Try this with your hands just a little forwards of your shoulder joints to give you more range.

CHALLENGES & BENEFITS

• Challenges your ability to control your neutral spine and pelvic positions.

• Mobilises spine, hips and shoulder joints.

• Loads the wrists and hips; improving bone density.

WATCHPOINTS

As for Cat, plus:

• When you move back with the spine extended in its reverse C-Curve, your lower back will round naturally; this is inevitable. But take care not to overly round your lower back as you move backwards.

• Keep the arms fully lengthened but avoid locking out (hyperextending the elbows).

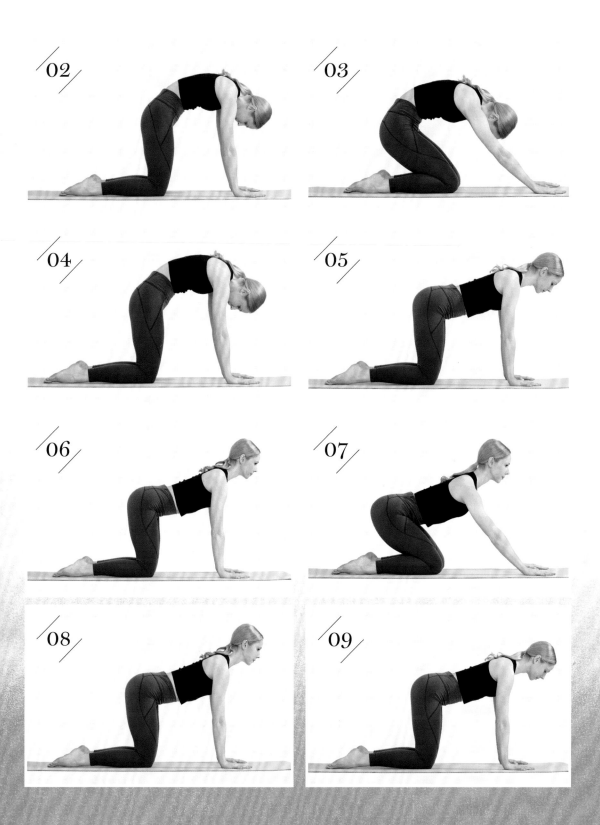

EXERCISE

Table Top Variations

Here we have taken the humble Table Top and elevated it to new heights by adding a string of new challenges!

STARTING POSITION

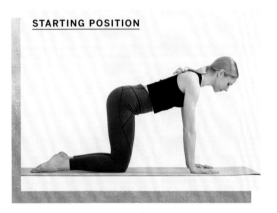

All the Table Top variations start in Four-point Kneeling (page 44).

Table Top Taps

Extra work for your gluteal muscles here. Note the immediately direction.

ACTION

01/ Breathe in to prepare.

02/ Breathe out as you slide one leg behind you, directly in line with your hip. Do not disturb the pelvis or spine.

03/ Breathe in as you lengthen and lift your leg to hip height, without moving anything else.

04/ Breathe out as you lower your foot down to the floor, but, and here's the difference, this time do not rest there, immediately...

05/ Breathe in and lift the leg to hip height.

Repeat the lift and lower leg x 5 without any change to the rest of your body. After 5 taps, return the foot to the floor and slide it back in.

Repeat with the other leg.

You can repeat the sequence twice. If you lose the breathing pattern, just continue to breathe normally.

CHALLENGES & BENEFITS

• Challenges, and therefore improves, your core stability.

• Challenges your ability to maintain neutral pelvis and spine while moving the legs and your balance.

• Mobilises the hips, encouraging lymph flow.

• Works the gluteal muscles, arms and shoulders.

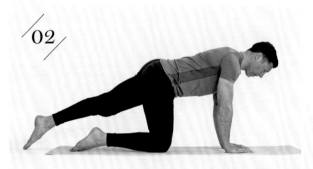

/02/

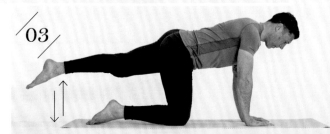

/03/

Table Top Leg Stretch

Here the action of the leg is very similar to the classical Single Leg Stretch, although, of course, you are in a totally different Starting Position!

Follow directions 1–3 above.

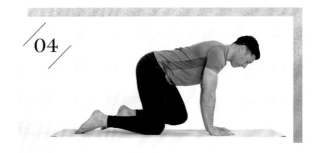

04/ Breathe out and then, as you breathe in, fold the leg in, bending the knee. Once again, focus on moving only the leg; everything else stays still. The challenge will be to not round your lower back as the knee folds in towards the chest.

05/ Breathe out as you straighten the leg again to hip height.

Repeat this folding and straightening of the leg x 5, before lowering the leg to the floor and repeating the sequence with the other leg.

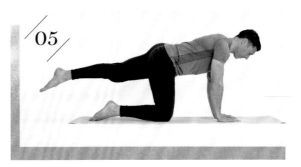

Table Top Leg Circles

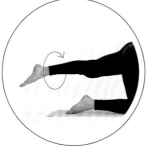

In this variation, you are asked to circle the leg – the size of the circle will depend on your flexibility and control. Start small, maybe the size of an apple, working up to a watermelon, providing you can still keep your pelvis and spine stable. The centre of your circle should be at the level of your hip.

Use The Hundred (page 176) breathing pattern here.

Follow Action Points 1–3 above, then:

04/ Circle your leg around. Do five circles one way on an out-breath, five circles the other way on an in-breath.

05/ Lower the leg and slide it back in with control, before repeating on the other side.

Repeat, alternating the legs twice, then return to the Starting Position.

WATCHPOINTS

• Use appropriate core connection to control your alignment and movements.

• Keep lengthening the spine from both ends. Think long and strong.

• Keep the active leg in line with your hip. You can lift your leg higher, providing you do not disturb your pelvis and spine.

• Check you are wide and open across your shoulders.

Moving on... Once you are proficient at the above versions, try the Table Top Taps with one arm lifted in front to shoulder height. Do not forget to lift the opposite arm to the active leg or you'll end up doing a one-sided wheelie! Warning: this is very challenging for both your stability and your balance!

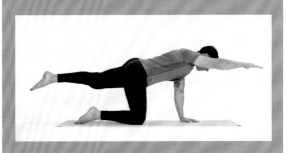

EXERCISE

Full Star

A valuable exercise that works the whole body.

STARTING POSITION

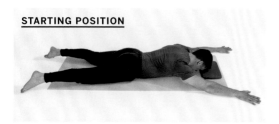

Prone (page 48). Your pelvis and lumbar spine are in neutral. Have your legs slightly wider than hip-width and turned out from the hips. Your arms are reaching above you, resting on the mat, slightly wider than shoulder-width, palms down.

ACTION

01/ Breathe in to prepare.

02/ Breathe out as you sequentially lift your head, neck and upper spine into Dart position (page 119). Ribs stay down. Shine your breastbone forwards and up.

03/ Breathe in and lengthen through the spine.

04/ Breathe out as you lengthen and lift opposite arm and leg slightly off the mat without disturbing your spine or pelvis.

05/ Breathe in as you lower your arm and leg back to the mat, keeping your upper back extension.

06/ Breathe out as you lift the other arm and leg.

Repeat up to x 10, alternating arms and legs. Then, with all limbs grounded, lengthen the spine back down to the Starting Position.

CHALLENGES & BENEFITS

• Challenges your core stability.

• Mobilises spine, shoulders and hips.

• Strengthens your upper back, shoulder and gluteal muscles.

• Reverses hunched posture.

• 'Opens' your hips.

• Encourages lymph flow.

WATCHPOINTS

• Use appropriate core connection to control your alignment and movements.

• Take care not to tip your head back – it stays in line with the spine.

• Do not over-reach with your arms; keep the width across your shoulders and the distance between your ears and shoulders.

• Lift your arm and leg only as high as you can maintain a still and stable pelvis and spine.

VARIATION:

Turn the palms to face each other if this is more comfortable for your shoulders.

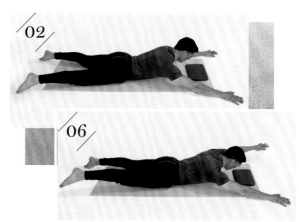

EXERCISE

Single Leg Pull Front Prep

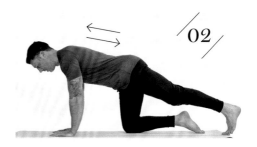

This is a variation of Front Leg Pull Prep. It is a fabulous end-of-the-day exercise. Do not think of this as a 'holding' exercise; it is not a plank, it is about building strength by controlling your alignment and movement.

STARTING POSITION

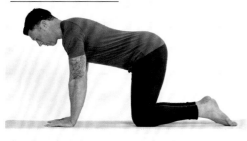

Four-point Kneeling (page 44).

ACTION

01/ Breathe in to prepare.

02/ Breathe out and slide your left leg along the mat in line with your hip joint. Tuck your toes under and take the weight onto the ball of the foot. Your trunk stays stable, but you may need to transfer your weight a little to stay centred.

03/ Breathe in and press back through your heels; your whole body will simultaneously shift backwards. Stay in one long line from head to heels. Stay central, do not allow the trunk to rotate.

04/ Breathe out as you bring your weight forwards again, and return your shoulders to directly over your wrists.

Repeat moving your body back and forth, in a long line x 4.

05/ Then, breathe in as you bend your knee, sliding the foot back to the Starting Position.

06/ Breathe out and repeat with the right leg.

Work up to repeating the above sequence x 3, alternating which leg you start with.

CHALLENGES & BENEFITS

• Challenges your core stability and control of alignment, especially preventing unwanted rotation.

• Mobilises the shoulders, hips and ankles.

• Gives a wonderful stretch to the legs!

• Strengthens legs, shoulders and arms.

WATCHPOINTS

• Use appropriate core connection to control your alignment and movements.

• You will probably need to turn your Dimmer Switch up (page 59) to avoid your pelvis and spine dipping down to one side.

• As you press your heel to the mat, continue to lengthen out through the crown of your head.

• Keep your shoulder blades connected to the back of your ribcage. Lift the weight of your body away from your arms and keep your chest open.

Side-kick Series: Front *and* Back

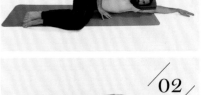

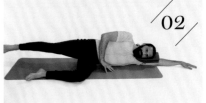

This is another fantastic exercise to do at the end of the day, when your hips might feel stiff.

STARTING POSITION

Lie on your left side, in a straight line; shoulders, hips and ankles stacked. Stretch your left arm out in line with your body and use a flat cushion or folded towel to keep your head aligned with your spine. Place your right hand on the mat in front of your ribcage and bend the elbow to lightly support you.

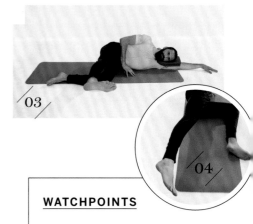

ACTION

01/ Breathe in to prepare.

02/ Breathe out and lengthen and lift your top leg back to be in line with your spine.

03/ Breathe in as you sweep your right leg forwards, hinging from the hip joint. The pelvis and spine remain stable. As you reach the end of the movement forwards, draw your leg slightly back, flex the foot and then pulse it a little further forwards.

04/ Breathe out as you point your foot and sweep the leg back, again to extend it just behind the hip joint.

Repeat up to x 10 before turning over onto the other side.

CHALLENGES & BENEFITS

• Challenges your core stability and balance.

• Mobilises your hips (encouraging lymph flow) and ankles.

• Stretches and strengthens your legs and works your waist muscles.

WATCHPOINTS

• Use appropriate core connection to control your alignment and movements.

• Keep both sides of your waist lengthened, and lifted.

• Keep your chest, and your gaze directly ahead of you.

• Your leg moves in isolation to the rest of your body. Do not disturb the pelvis or spine.

• The movement of the leg should be brisk but controlled.

• Keep the underneath leg active; this will help you balance.

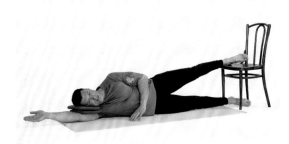

EXERCISE

Chair Lifts

It is surprising how using the chair really helps you to lengthen your whole body out.

STARTING POSITION

Lie on your side in a straight line. Have your top foot resting on the seat of a sturdy chair. Your underneath arm is stretched out in a line with your body. Place your other hand at chest level in front of you for support. Your underneath leg can be in parallel or turned out from the hip, foot pointed or flexed.

/ 02 /

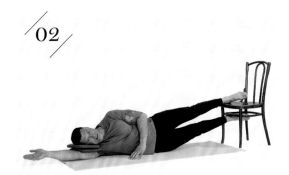

ACTION

01/ Breathe in to prepare.

02/ Breathe out as you lengthen and lift the underneath leg as far as you can without disturbing the pelvis (or the chair!).

03/ Breathe in and lower the leg, but not all the way to the mat, then lift it again immediately.

Repeat up to x 10 on this side, then repeat on the other side.

CHALLENGES & BENEFITS

• Challenges your core stability and balance.

• Mobilises your hips.

• Works the waist strongly and the inner thighs.

VARIATION

Use ankle weights of up to 1kg (2lb 4 oz) each weight. It is a good idea to alternate - legs parallel, turned out, feet pointed, feet flexed each time you do a workout.

WATCHPOINTS

• Use appropriate core connection to control your alignment and movements.

• Keep your waist lengthened and lifted equally on both sides.

• If your foot is flexed, really lengthen through the heel.

• Keep your upper body squarely facing forwards; pelvis and spine still.

EXERCISE

The Pilates Squat

This is becoming a staple in our classes and is an essential part of Sit to Stand and Stand to Sit (pages 190–3). Once the basic Squat is mastered, play with added challenges.

CHALLENGES & BENEFITS

• Challenges your control of the alignment of head, ribs, pelvis and lower limbs.

• Mobilises hips, knees, ankles and shoulders.

• Works thighs, calves and gluteal muscles.

WATCHPOINTS

• Use appropriate core connection to control your alignment and movements.

• Do not squat too low; avoid taking your bottom below knee level.

• Check your leg alignment. Send the knees directly forwards, not in or out. Check that your ankles are not rolling in or out.

• Ensure equal weight between both legs.

• Use your gluteals to bring you back upright.

• Keep all your toes on the floor.

• For this version, keep the heels on the floor throughout.

• Pelvis and spine remain neutral.

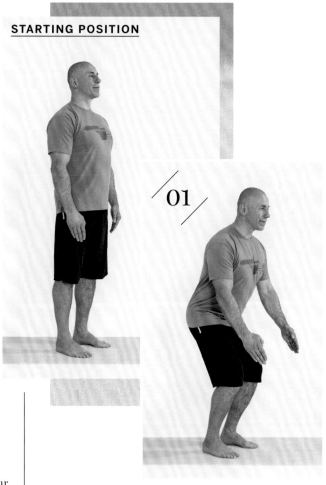

STARTING POSITION

01

STARTING POSITION

Stand tall on the floor, not on your mat. Arms lengthened by your sides, palms facing inwards.

ACTION

01/ Breathe in and bend your hips, knees and ankles into a small squat. You will naturally hinge forwards from your hips but keep your spine straight. Your arms may reach forwards to help you balance.

02/ Breathe out as you straighten up tall.

Repeat up to x 10.

EXERCISE

Walking *on the* Spot Squat

A great variation to do outdoors if you can find level ground. You can wear flexible soled shoes.

STARTING POSITION

Stand tall on a firm level surface. Arms lengthened by your sides, palms facing inwards.

ACTION

01/ Breathe in and bend your hips, knees and ankles into a small squat.

02/ Stay squatted and breathe normally as you raise both heels.

03/ Then lower one heel to establish a walking on the spot action.

04/ Walk in the squat before stopping walking.

05/ Straighten back up tall.

Repeat up to x 4.

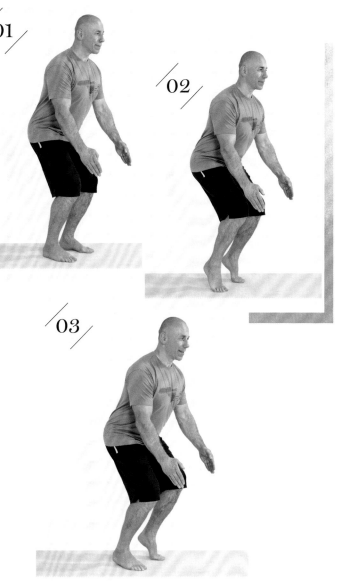

CHALLENGES & BENEFITS

As for Squats, plus:

• Challenges your co-ordination.

WATCHPOINTS

As for Squats (opposite), plus:

• Swing your arms with ease; staying wide and open across your collarbones.

• Keep good alignment of the hips, knees and ankles – glance down to check your knees and ankles are directed forwards and not rolling in or out.

• Remind your gluteal muscles that they need to work to straighten you back up.

EXERCISE

Ski Squats

You can layer on the challenges here. This always makes me think of Eddie the Eagle.

STARTING POSITION

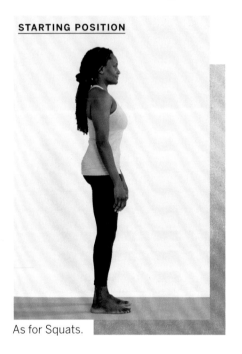

As for Squats.

ACTION

01/ Breathe in and bend your hips, knees and ankles into a small squat. Simultaneously, bring your arms behind you (as if skiing downhill).

02/ Breathe out as you come upright.

03/ Breathe in now as you come up onto your toes.

04/ Breathe out as you lower your heels, coming back down into a Squat.

Repeat up to x 6 heel raises before returning back to upright.

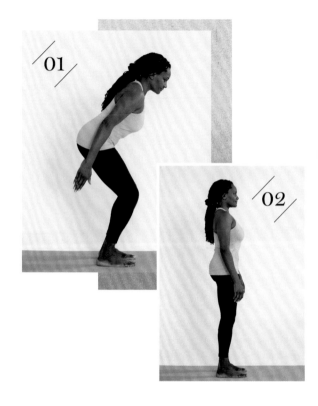

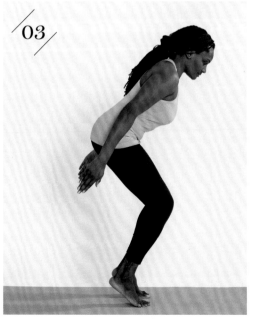

CHALLENGES & BENEFITS

As for squats, plus:

• Challenges and improves balance.

WATCHPOINTS

As for squats, plus:

• Use appropriate core connection to control your alignment and movements.

• Take care to keep control of your alignment head to toes.

• If you can, keep your weight on the balls of your feet as you Squat initially (but keep your heels down); that will help you transfer the weight as you come up onto your toes.

• Once again, cue your gluteal muscles to work as you come back upright.

Layering on new challenges to your squats
You could try...

01/ Adding a Ribcage Closure (page 73) or Arm Circles (page 76) to your Squat.

02/ Staying up on your toes and balancing for a few breaths.

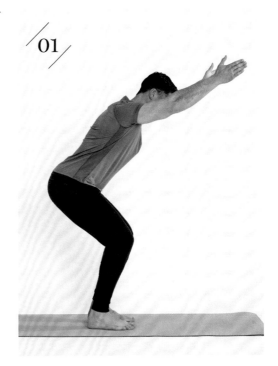

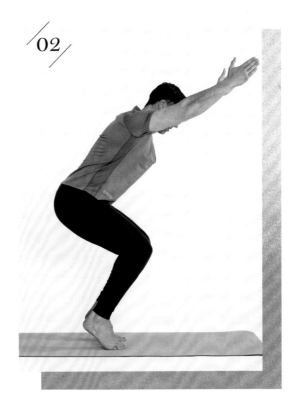

Exercises for *Strength* and *Flexibility*

In this chapter we will introduce you to some of the more challenging exercises. Truthfully, nearly every exercise in this book works on your strength and flexibility, however, we have singled these out as particularly challenging. The good news is that the more challenging they are, the greater the benefits when you master them. We will be interspersing the exercises into many of your workouts (pages 179–97), not just the Strength and Flexibility ones. Obviously, if you are not ready to do them yet, leave them out.

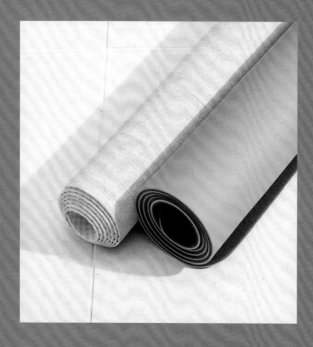

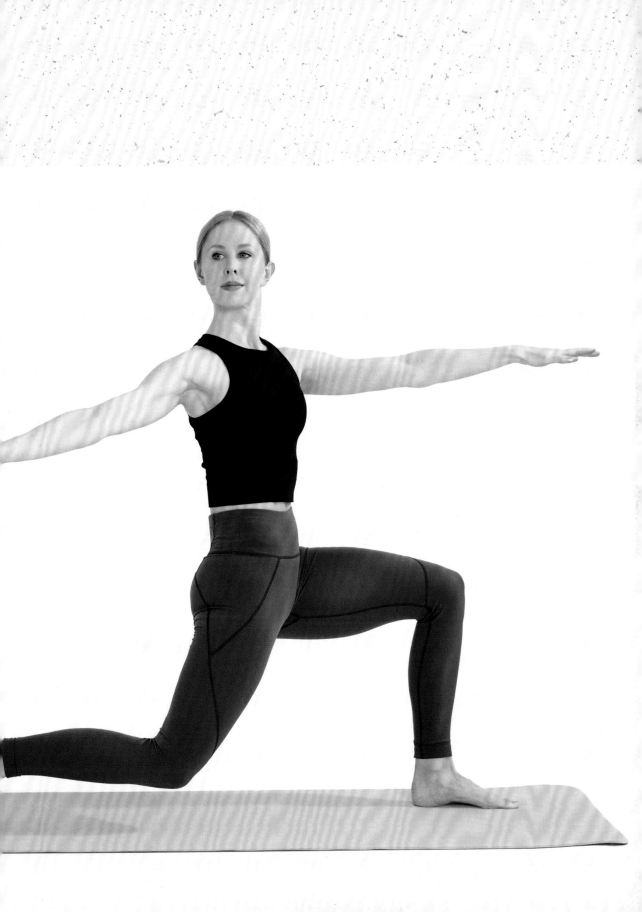

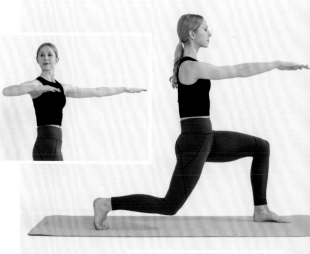

EXERCISE

Static Lunge Variations

Holding a Static Lunge position (page 53) is not easy, so only try a few repetitions initially and build up strength.

• <u>Bow and Arrow page 87</u>

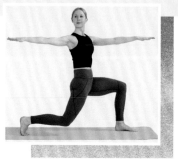

STARTING POSITION

Stand tall, feet hip-width apart and in parallel. Step forwards with your right/left foot, bending the right/left knee and right/left hip to about 90 degrees, while simultaneously bending the left/right knee to as near to parallel as possible. Stay as upright as possible.

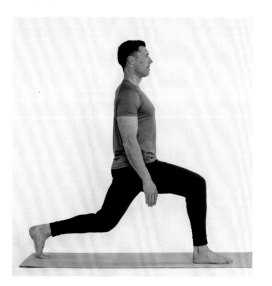

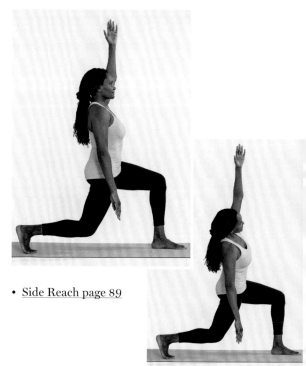

THEN, WE CAN ADD A VARIETY OF ADDITIONAL CHALLENGES:

• <u>Side Reach page 89</u>

When you have competed the Actions, return to Starting Position with control, then repeat bringing the other foot forwards.

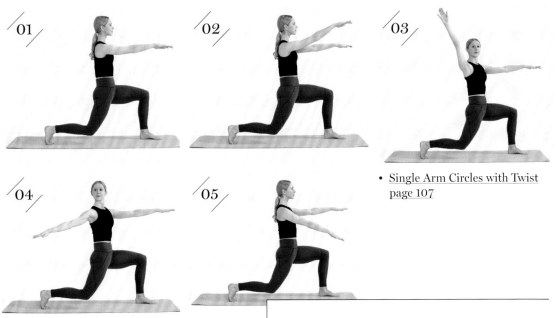

01 02 03

04 05

- <u>Single Arm Circles with Twist page 107</u>

- <u>Waist Twist page 85</u>

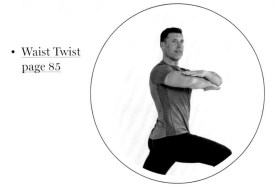

- <u>Chest Expansion page 104</u>

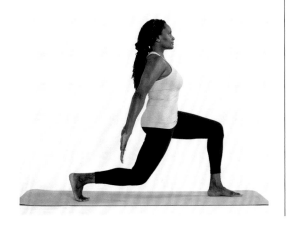

CHALLENGES & BENEFITS

These vary according to the variation. In addition to challenging your ability to control your alignment top to toe, holding a Lunge position also challenges, and therefore improves, your endurance.

- Challenges your core stability and alignment.

- Challenges your balance and co-ordination.

- Mobilises your hips, knees and ankles.

SHARED WATCHPOINTS

- Use appropriate core connection to control your alignment and movements.

- Step out as far as you can maintain good alignment; much will depend on your stability and flexibility.

- Double check that your pelvis and spine stay in neutral and you stay as vertical (Centreline) as possible.

- Front leg: knee stays above ankle and in line with your second toe.

- Back leg: knee is bent and heel lifted.

EXERCISE

Split Stance 'Curtsy' Squats

Just in case you meet royalty!

CHALLENGES & BENEFITS

• Challenges, and thus improves, your ability to control your trunk and lower limb alignment.

• Challenges and improves your core stability.

• Challenges your balance and co-ordination.

• Mobilises hips, knees, ankles and feet.

• Works gluteal, thigh and calf muscles.

STARTING POSITION

Stand tall in a wide Pilates Stance (page 51), legs turned out from the hips.

ACTION

01/ Breathe in and check your alignment.

02/ Breathe out and step back with one foot to 'curtsy' and squat; the back heel will be lifted, both knees will bend as you curtsy.

03/ Breathe in and step back to the Starting Position, before repeating with the other leg.

Repeat up to x 6.

Or... stay in the Curtsy Squat position and dip a few times before stepping back forwards.

STARTING POSITION

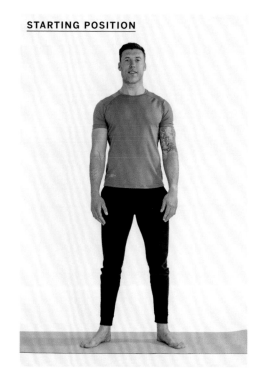

/02/

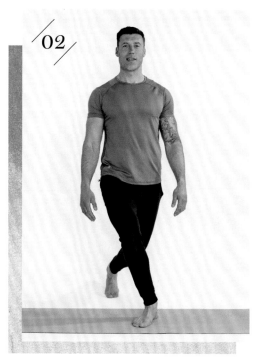

With Floating Arms

This elevates the Curtsy Squat to a full body exercise, adding an aerobic benefit. As you step back float both arms up (as for Floating Arms, page 74). Bring your arms down as you step forwards.

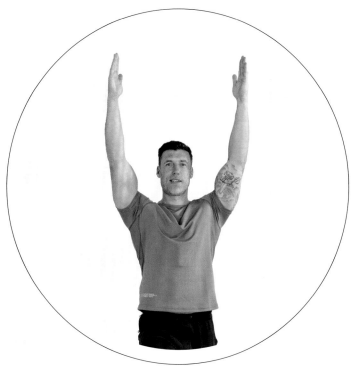

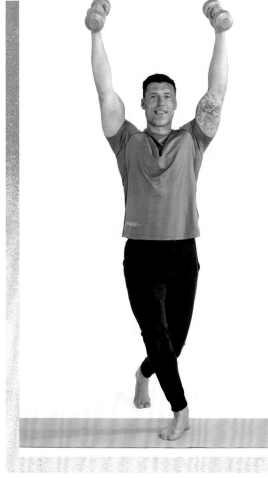

CHALLENGES & BENEFITS

As opposite, plus:

• Mobilises your shoulders and raises your heart rate.

WATCHPOINTS

• Use appropriate core connection to control your alignment and movements.

• Leg alignment is crucial here. Normally, we ask you to keep your gaze forwards as you squat but, just this once, as you squat glance down and briefly check that your knees are bending over your second toes.

• Keep control of your head, ribcage and pelvic alignment – they stay stacked as you dip.

• Try to return to the same Starting Position if you can.

• Do not dip too low; it is a small squat not a full-blown deep curtsy!

EXERCISE

Dynamic Lunges

and Fun Variations

Following on from Curtsy Squats, these Dynamic Lunges and their variations add a cardiovascular element to your workouts. Please do not forget to apply your Fundamentals to these Lunges. If necessary, do them super slow until you are confident that you are in control.

STARTING POSITION

Stand tall, feet hip-width apart and in parallel. Double check that your pelvis and spine are in neutral.

ACTION

01/ Breathe in as you step forwards with your right foot, bending the right knee and right hip to about 90 degrees, while simultaneously extending the left hip and bending the left knee parallel to the floor. As your right hip flexes, your torso may naturally lean forwards slightly. Your left heel will lift to allow you to stay upright.

02/ Breathe out as you straighten the right leg and step back to the Starting Position.

Repeat up to x 6 with each leg.

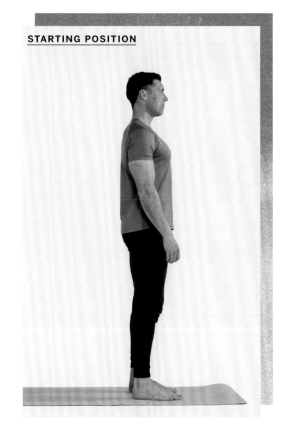

STARTING POSITION

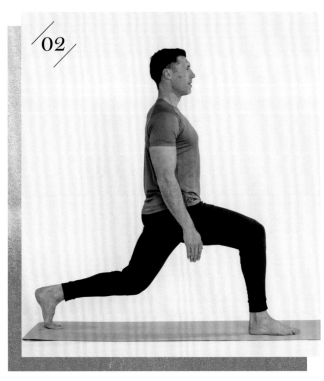

/02/

Dynamic Backwards Lunge

Some people find this easier, others harder... simply follow the directions above but step backwards!

ADDING CHALLENGES

As for Curtsy Squats, we want to keep the Lunges flowing so it is best to simply add actions such as:

• Ribcage Closure

• Floating Arms with or without weights.

CHALLENGES & BENEFITS

As for Curtsy Squats.

WATCHPOINTS

• Use appropriate core connection to control your alignment and movements.

• Bend your knees as far as you can while staying in control. It is better to do a good mini lunge than a bad deep one!

• Stay aware of the relationship between your head, ribcage, and pelvis.

• Remain as upright as possible; long and strong through your spine.

• Ensure that the knee of the leg stepping forwards does not go beyond the toes and stays centred over the foot.

• Check that your knees and ankles do not roll in or out.

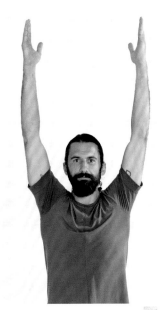

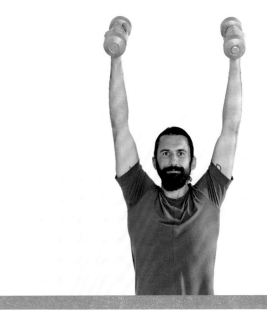

EXERCISE

High-kneeling Advanced Side Reach

This challenging version of Side Reach has the perfect balance of working on both your strength and flexibility. Depending on your flexibility, you may (or may not) feel a strong stretch in your inner thighs. It is a good idea to ensure you are 'warmed up' before you try it. Exercises such as Knee Openings (page 63) and Chair Lifts (page 149) will suitably mobilise your hip joints and Squats (page 150) and Lunges (page 160) will warm you up nicely.

Note that you will be able to side flex more in the opposite direction to your straightened leg.

STARTING POSITION

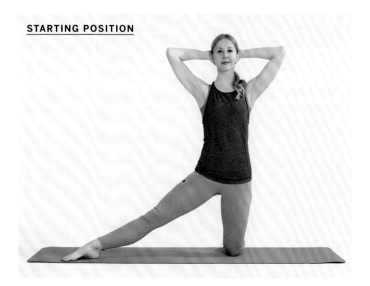

High Kneeling (page 46). Start with the legs hip-width apart, then take your right leg out to the side, slightly in front of your hip. Point the foot in line with your leg or bring the foot to face forwards (one will probably feel more natural). Float your arms up and place them behind your head.

CHALLENGES & BENEFITS

• Challenges your balance; plus pelvic and core stability.

• Challenges your control of alignment.

• Mobilises the spine into side flexion.

• Mobilises hips, shoulders and (depending on foot position) ankles.

• Promotes flexibility in the upper spine and ribcage and aids breathing.

WATCHPOINTS

• Use appropriate core connection to control your alignment and movements.

• Do not force the side flexion; even a small amount is beneficial.

• Keep your hips square to the front.

ACTION

01/ Breathe in to prepare.

02/ Breathe out as you reach your head, neck and upper spine up and over to the left. Direct your elbow in an arc up and to the ceiling.

03/ Breathe into your open side.

04/ Breathe out as you restack the spine to come upright.

05/ Breathe in wide.

06/ Breathe out as you side bend sequentially over to the other side.

07/ Breathe into the open side.

08/ Breathe out and return upright.

09/ Breathe in to bring the arms down.

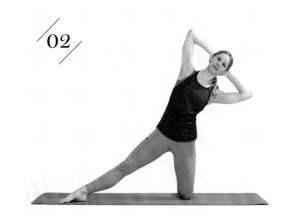

02/

05/

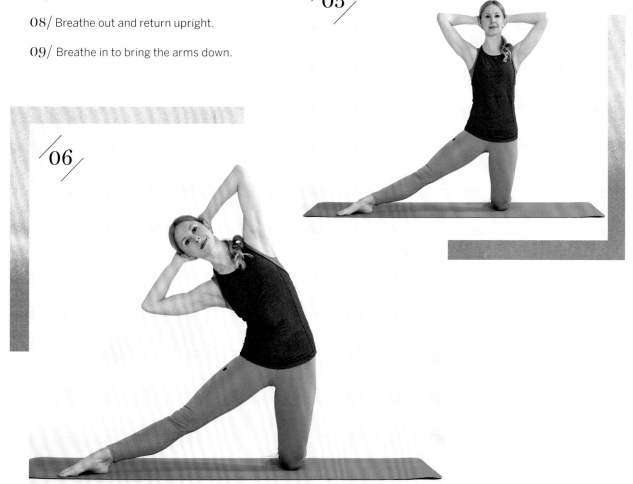

06/

EXERCISE

The Back Bridge

This is proving to be a very popular exercise and is great to do at the end of the day as it really opens out your hips and shoulders.

STARTING POSITION

Sit tall on the mat with your knees bent in front of you, hip-width apart, feet flat on the floor. Have your hands down by your sides in line with your shoulders, palms flat on the mat, fingers facing forwards. Depending on the length of your arms and body, you may need to have your elbows slightly bent. Ensure that you are in a lengthened position and your shoulders are open.

ACTION

01/ Breathe in to prepare.

02/ Breathe out and lift your bottom up from the mat, sending your hips to the ceiling, knees forwards.

03/ Breathe in and hold this position.

04/ Breathe out and lower with control.

Repeat up to x 8.

CHALLENGES & BENEFITS

• Challenges your scapular, lumbar and pelvic stability.

• Works your gluteal, shoulder and arm muscles.

• Mobilises and opens the hips and shoulders.

WATCHPOINTS

• Use appropriate core connection to control your alignment and movements.

• Keep your body in a 'straight' line – do not drop your bottom down.

• Keep lengthening up through the crown of your head. Do not be tempted to sink into your shoulders.

STARTING POSITION

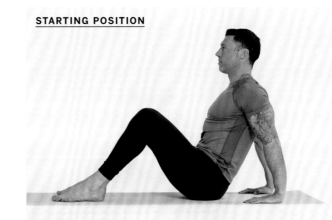

/02/

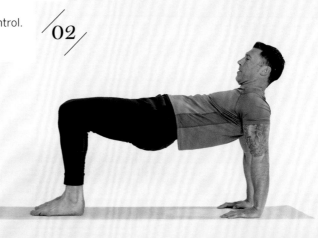

Back Bridge with Dips

Like Side Press-ups, these are very powerful exercises for the arms and upper body.

ACTION

Follow Action Points 1–2 above, then:

03/ Slowly and with control, breathe in and bend your elbows backwards to dip down. Take care not to sink between your shoulders. Your elbows will probably only bend slightly.

04/ Breathe out and straighten your elbows.

Repeat up to x 8 before lowering the body down.

CHALLENGES & BENEFITS

As for Back Bridge, plus:

• Mobilises the elbows and works upper arm muscles.

WATCHPOINTS

• Maintain the distance between your ears and your shoulders.

• Collarbones stay wide and open.

• Keep lengthening through the spine.

/03/

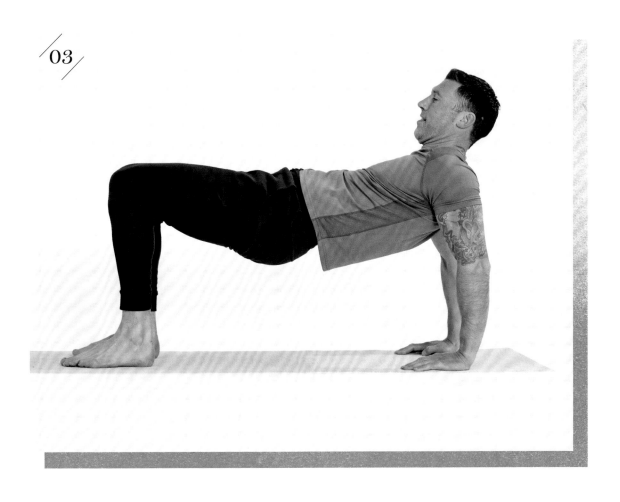

EXERCISE

Dart *into* Star

Here we are combining two of our favourite back strengthening exercises to ensure you are posture perfect.

STARTING POSITION

Prone (page 48). Have your legs shoulder-width apart and turned out from the hips. Arms lengthened by your sides, palms either up or down, whichever feels more comfortable.

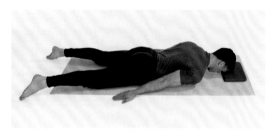

ACTION

01/ Breathe in to prepare.

02/ Breathe out as you extend the upper spine, lengthening and lifting first your head, then neck and upper spine, one vertebra at a time.

03/ Breathe in and float one arm up out to the side and above you. Let it float up, following its natural arc, and then allow it to rest on the floor.

04/ Breathe out and repeat with the other arm so that you create an 'X' shape.

05/ Breathe in as you lengthen and lift opposite arm and leg away from you.

06/ Breathe out and return the arm and leg.

Repeat x 5, alternating opposite arm and leg, then:

07/ With the spine still lifted, breathe in and float one arm back down by your side.

08/ Breathe out and float the other arm back down.

09/ Breathe in as you lengthen and lower the spine back down.

Repeat up to x 3.

CHALLENGES & BENEFITS

• Challenges you to extend your spine sequentially and maintain the extension.

• The added limb actions challenge your pelvic stability and strength.

• Works your back, gluteal, shoulder and arm muscles.

• Mobilises your upper spine, hips, shoulders and arms

WATCHPOINTS

As for Dart (page 119), plus:

• Use appropriate core connection to control your alignment and movements.

• Try not to press down on your arms as you extend your back.

• Raise your leg only as high as you can without disturbing the pelvis and spine.

• Fully lengthen your legs but avoid locking knees.

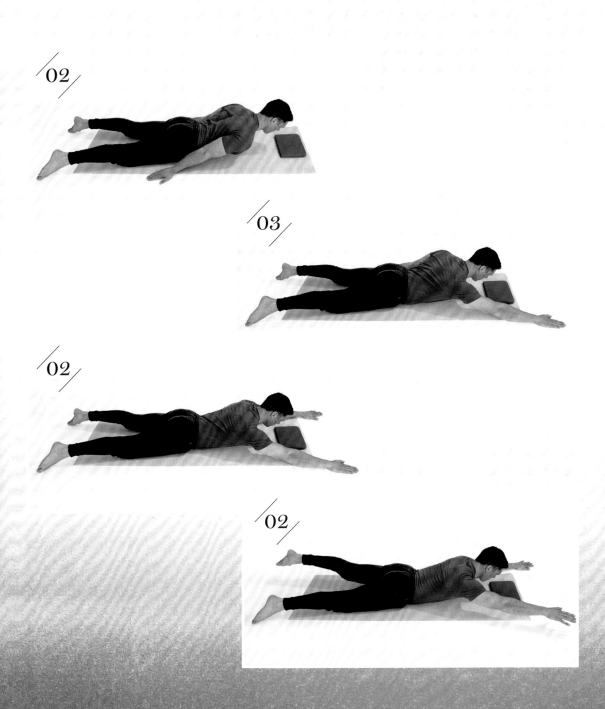

EXERCISE

Cobra Prep

with Arm Slide and Single Heel Kick

More multitasking. Refresh your memory of Cobra Prep on page 168. Lots of directions, lots of benefits.

STARTING POSITION

Prone (page 48), rest your forehead on the mat. Your legs are straight, slightly wider than hip-width and turned out from the hips. Bend your elbows and position your hands slightly wider than, and just above, shoulder height. Make sure that your shoulders are released, and collarbones are wide.

ACTION

01/ Breathe in to prepare.

02/ Breathe out as you lengthen and lift your head and then your chest off the mat. Your lower ribs remain in contact with the mat, open your chest and focus on directing it forwards.

03/ Breathe in and slide one hand forwards along the floor.

04/ Breathe out, slide the arm back.

05/ Breathe in and slide the other hand forwards.

06/ Breathe out and slide it back.

07/ Breathe in as you return your chest and head sequentially down to the mat.

08/ Breathe out as you bend one knee to do two small, brisk pulsing 'kicks', pointing your foot towards the centre of your buttock.

09/ Breathe in as you straighten the leg.

10/ Breathe out as you repeat two small, brisk pulsing kicks but this time flexing your ankle in.

11/ Repeat the bending, pointing, flexing with the other leg.

Repeat the Heel Kicks twice with each leg, then repeat the whole sequence once more, restarting from Action Point 1.

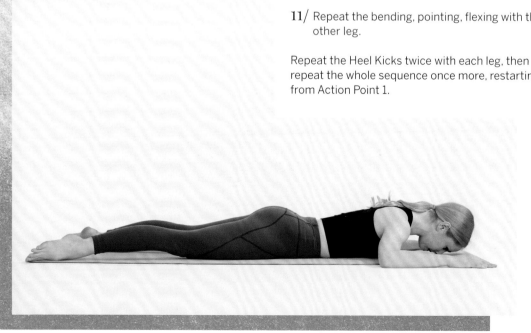

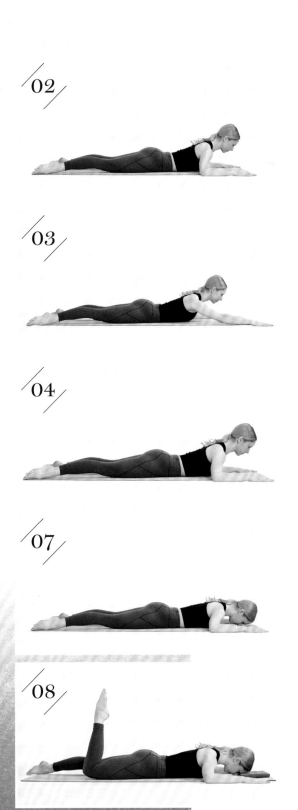

02

03

04

07

08

CHALLENGES & BENEFITS

• Challenges your ability to extend the upper spine sequentially with control.

• Challenges your pelvic and scapular stability.

• Challenges your co-ordination.

• Mobilises the upper spine, helping to promote better posture and breathing.

• Works your back muscles.

• Mobilises your knees and ankles.

WATCHPOINTS

As for Cobra Prep (page 168), plus:

• Use appropriate core connection to control your alignment and movements.

• The key to this combination exercise is to maintain stability in your trunk throughout.

• Only slide the hand as far as you can without disturbing your back extension.

• This leg action is very similar to the Single Heel Kick. Try to achieve the same fluid, pulsing action and try not to disturb your alignment.

• Try not to lock out your knee as you extend it.

EXERCISE

Full Cobra

The ultimate back exercise, and the perfect way to balance any abdominal work. Practise Cobra Prep (page 168) to prepare for Full Cobra.

STARTING POSITION

Prone (page 48). Rest your forehead on the mat or a folded towel. Your legs are straight, slightly wider than hip-width and turned out from the hips. Bend your elbows and position your hands just wider than your shoulders and just above them. Your shoulders are released and your collarbones wide.

ACTION

01/ Breathe in to prepare.

02/ Breathe out as you lengthen the front of the neck to roll and lift your head and continue to smoothly peel the front of the body off the mat. First the breastbone, then the ribcage and the abdominal area and finally the front of your pelvis. As the body wheels off the mat, your arms will begin to straighten. Continue to lengthen the legs behind the body.

03/ Breathe in and hold the extended back position.

04/ Breathe out as you lower the spine down sequentially; first the front of your pelvis, then the abdominal area, the ribcage, breastbone and finally the head.

Repeat up to x 6 before coming up into Four-point Kneeling (page 44). Bring your feet together and fold back into the Rest Position (page 98) to release your spine.

CHALLENGES & BENEFITS

• Challenges your ability to extend the spine sequentially with stability.

• Mobilises your spine, hips, elbows and shoulders.

• Works your back and arm muscles.

WATCHPOINTS

• Use appropriate core connection to control your alignment and movements.

• Do not just think about the back of your body when doing this exercise. You also need to lengthen the front of your body.

• At the height of the Full Cobra, allow your hips to open and the front of your pelvis to lose contact with the mat.

• Your arms may not fully straighten; this depends on the length of your spine and arms, as well as your flexibility.

• Keep your legs on the mat, reaching away from you throughout.

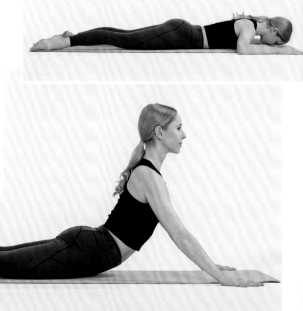

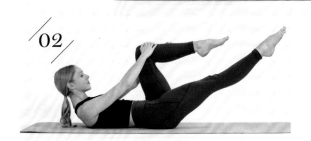

Single Leg Stretch

The full classical version remains one of the ultimate abdominal exercises.

STARTING POSITION

Relaxation Position (page 37). Double Knee Fold (page 65) one leg at a time with stability. Keeping your heels connected and your feet softly pointed, open your knees slightly.

Breathe in to prepare. As you breathe out, nod your head, and sequentially wheel your neck and upper body off the mat into a Curl Up (page 84). Lengthen your arms forwards and place your hands on the outside of your shins.

ACTION

01/ Breathe into the back of your ribcage.

02/ Breathe out as you straighten your left leg forwards in line with the hip. Simultaneously place the left hand on the right knee and gently draw the right leg in towards your torso.

03/ Continue to breathe out as you switch legs, bending the left leg in and drawing it in towards your torso as you press the right leg away. Your right hand will now be positioned on the left knee and the outside of the left shin bone.

04/ Breathe in as you repeat a further two leg stretches, pressing your legs away in turn.

Repeat up to x 5 before bringing both knees in towards your torso. Then roll back down to the mat. With stability, return your feet to the mat, one at a time.

CHALLENGES & BENEFITS

• Challenges your core stability and ability to control your leg alignment.

• Mobilises your spine, hips and knees.

• Builds stamina and endurance.

WATCHPOINTS

• Use appropriate core connection to control your alignment and movements.

• Keep all your movements controlled, smooth and flowing.

• Pelvis remains undisturbed throughout; if necessary, stretch the leg away higher.

• Stay curled up. Use your arms to draw your legs towards you and not to pull your spine up further.

• Keep your focus down onto your abdominal area.

• Keep your shoulders and neck free from tension.

• Keep a slight turn-out of both legs throughout.

EXERCISE

Prep *for the* Hundred *and* Roll Up

The reason this exercise is in this section is that it requires you to stay curled up for a considerable time, while co-ordinating arms and legs so it makes an excellent preparation for classical Roll Ups and Hundreds. It would be wise to practise Curls Ups (page 84) before attempting this version. You may want to move to the bottom of your mat so that your feet slide easily.

STARTING POSITION

Relaxation Position (page 37) but with your arms lifted above your shoulders, palms facing away.

ACTION

01/ Breathe in to prepare.

02/ Breathe out as you nod your head and curl up, simultaneously pressing down both arms until they hover at hip height.

03/ Breathe into the back of your ribcage to help you curl up further, while sliding one leg away in line with your hip.

04/ Breathe out and slide the other leg away.

05/ Breathe in as you slide the first leg back.

06/ Breathe out and slide the second leg back.

07/ Breathe in and roll back down with control, simultaneously raising the arms up to the Starting Position.

Repeat up to x 6, alternating which leg you slide away first.

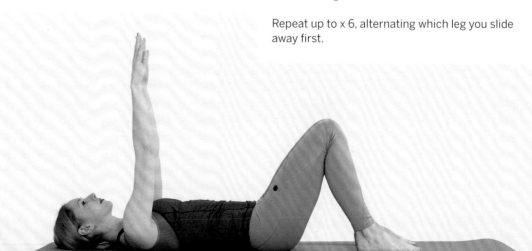

/02/

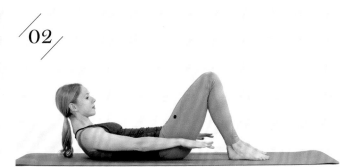

/03/

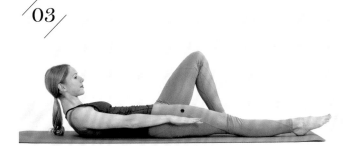

/04/

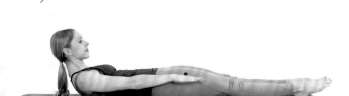

/06/

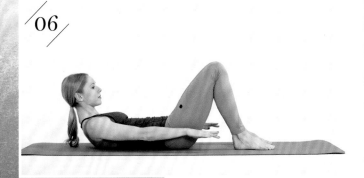

CHALLENGES & BENEFITS

• Challenges your spinal and pelvic stability.

• Challenges your stamina.

• Challenges your ability to control your alignment and co-ordination.

• Mobilises spine, shoulders, hips and knees.

• Works the abdominals, strongly.

WATCHPOINTS

• Use appropriate core connection to control your alignment and movements.

• Keep wide and open across your collarbones.

• Keep reaching through your fingertips throughout.

• There should be no tension in your neck. If there is, curl back down; it may be too challenging for you.

• When curled up, keep your gaze down towards your pubic bone.

• Your pelvis remains neutral.

• Check that you are sliding your legs in line with your hips.

EXERCISE

Roll Up

The best way to prepare for this exercise is to do Prep for the Hundred (page 172) and exercises where you roll through the spine: Spine Curls (page 78), Cat (page 80) and Roll Downs (page 93).

STARTING POSITION

Relaxation Position (page 37) but with both legs extended. They can be in parallel together or slightly apart. Feet flexed or softly pointed. Your pelvis and spine are in neutral. 'Ribcage Closure' (just created a new verb) your arms overhead to ear level.

ACTION

01/ Breathe in to prepare.

02/ Breathe out as you raise your arms and simultaneously begin to roll up from your head, neck and upper back. Continue to roll up through the rest of the spine, sequentially wheeling it off the mat, one vertebra at a time. Lengthen the C-Curved spine over your legs. Reach the arms forwards, ensuring they maintain their relationship with your neck and head.

03/ Breathe in as you begin to roll the pelvis and spine back down along the mat, ensuring that you initiate the movement from the pelvis.

03/ Breathe out as you continue to wheel the whole spine sequentially down onto the mat, returning the head and the arms on the final part of your exhalation.

Repeat up to x 5.

CHALLENGES & BENEFITS

• Challenges your core stability and abdominal strength.

• Challenges your ability to roll through your Centreline segmentally.

• Mobilises spine, hips and shoulders.

WATCHPOINTS

Lots we know, but this is a big exercise.

• Use appropriate core connection to control your alignment and movements.

• Roll smoothly through each segment of your spine. Do not roll forwards from your hips until the spine is fully flexed into an even C-Curve.

• Lengthen, lengthen, lengthen throughout.

• Roll directly through your Centreline, avoiding any deviations to either side.

• Keep a relationship between the shoulders and the back of your ribcage. Neither force them to depress, nor allow them to over-elevate, especially while reaching forwards over the legs.

• Focus on the control of the movement with your breath; keep the whole movement even and flowing.

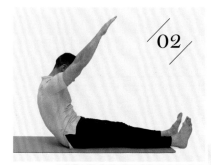

02

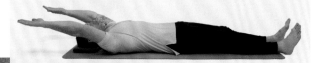

STARTING POSITION

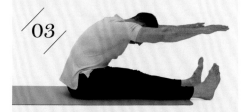

03

EXERCISE

Side Press-ups

In this exercise, you are using your body weight to tone your arms. This means that it is often easier for women than men, as men's upper body weight is usually considerably greater.

STARTING POSITION

Side Lying with your legs slightly bent, feet in line with your body. If you are lying on your left side, place your right hand on the floor in front of you, approximately chest level, palm down, fingers pointing in the direction of your head. You may have to adjust this hand position, depending on the length of your body so that you can get the right leverage to press up. Your left hand crosses your body and rests on your ribs.

ACTION

01/ Breathe in to prepare and lengthen through your body, head to tail.

02/ Breathe out as you press down through your hand, straightening the arm so that your upper body lifts. There will be a slight trunk rotation as you do so.

03/ Breathe in and hold the press up.

04/ Breathe out and slowly, with control, lower yourself down.

Repeat up to x 6 on each side.

CHALLENGES & BENEFITS

• Challenges you to lift your upper body against gravity, while maintaining good alignment.

• Works your arms, shoulders and waist.

WATCHPOINTS

• Use appropriate core connection to control your alignment and movements.

• Before you press up, try to connect to the muscles below your shoulder blades; the ones which wrap around your ribcage under your armpits, as these muscles help stabilise your shoulder blades.

• Keep control of your mid-section as you lift and lower.

• Keep lengthening through both sides of your waist.

• Your feet and knees remain down. You can adjust their position if that helps with the leverage.

STARTING POSITION

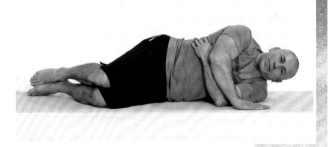

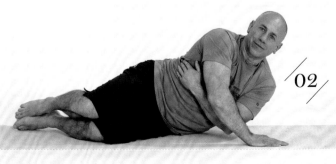

02/

The Hundred

This classical exercise is a fitting grand finale for the Pilates Express® programme. We have given you stages here, culminating in the full version. Please work through the stages carefully as each 'ups' the challenge. A fabulous way to energise the entire body and get the blood pumping.

Hundred Stage 1 Breathing

You will be delighted to know that you've learnt The Hundred Stage 1 (the breathing pattern) already on page 99. Here's a quick reminder.

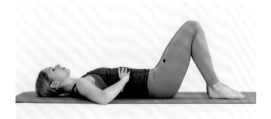

Hundred Stage 2

STARTING POSITION

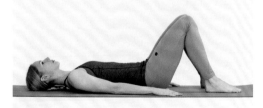

Relaxation Position (page 37).

ACTION

01/ Breathe in to prepare.

02/ Breathe out as you nod your head and curl up through the spine, raising the arms slightly off the mat.

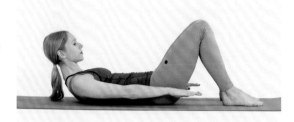

03/ Staying in Curl Up, start to beat your arms, breathing in for a count of five, out for a count of five. Repeat the beating and breathing up to x 10 (100 beats).

04/ Then 'still' the arms and breathe out as you curl back down.

Hundred Stage 3

This is identical to Stage 2 but your legs are now in a parallel Double Knee Fold (page 65).

STARTING POSITION

Relaxation Position (page 37). Double Knee Fold, one leg at a time, with stability. Connect your inner thighs so that the legs are together in parallel.

Then follow all the directions above, before rolling back down and returning the feet, one at a time, with stability, to the mat.

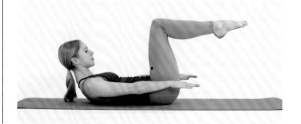

Hundred Stage 4

As for Stage 3, but as you Curl Up simultaneously straighten both legs to an angle of approximately 80 degrees from the mat.

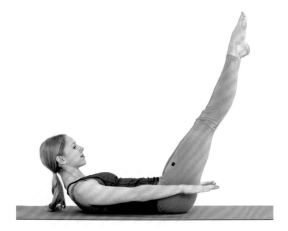

When you have finished your 100 beats, bend your knees, curl back down and safely return the feet to the floor, one at a time, with stability.

Hundred Stage 5

A fitting end to the programme. If ever you need an exercise to improve your overall health, breathing, immunity, even your heart health, the Hundred ticks every box.

Your Starting Position is slightly different here. You are in a Double Knee Fold (page 65) but your legs are turned out from the hips and toes are touching.

Follow the directions for Stage 4 but, as you straighten your legs, they will automatically come into a Pilates Stance turned-out position. Really connect your inner thighs as you do so.

CHALLENGES & BENEFITS

• Challenges your endurance, especially of your abdominal muscles!

• Improves your breathing and stamina.

• Mobilises spine, hips and shoulders.

• Lengthens the hamstrings (if you straighten the legs).

WATCHPOINTS

• Use appropriate core connection to control your alignment and movements.

• Really focus on maintaining your core connection; pelvis still and stable, whilst breathing wide into the back of your ribcage.

• Focus on your breathing, squeezing every bit of air out on the exhalations.

• Stay wide and open across your collarbones and shoulder blades.

• As you beat the arms, keep your gaze down on your pubic bone.

• Keep your arms straight and lengthened but be careful not to lock your elbows.

• Lengthen through your hands and fingers. The arm, wrist and hand move as one and the movement comes purely from your shoulder joint. No flapping wrists please.

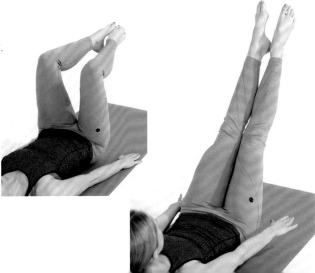

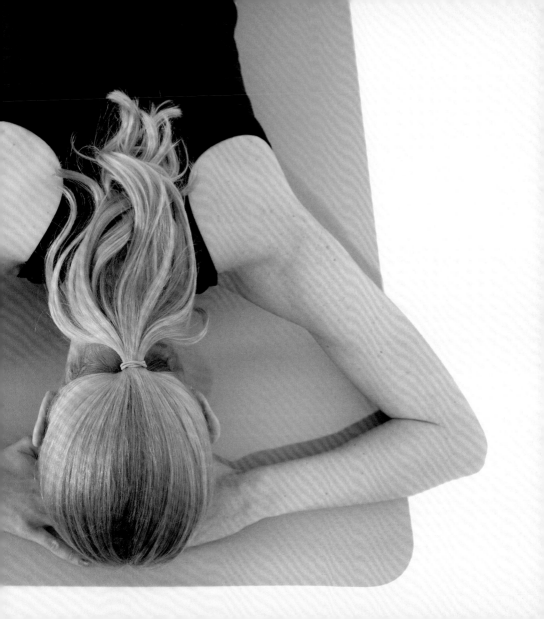

The *Pilates Express*® Workouts

CHAPTER TWO

The Pilates Express® Day

We are hoping that, by the time you reach this chapter, you are familiar with most of the exercises in the programme. We want our mini workouts to become habitual, daily rituals, as automatic and essential as brushing your teeth.

The coronavirus pandemic robbed us all of normality. For many of us, we lost the opportunity for the usual rituals that punctuated our working days. I, for one, keenly felt this loss. I first learnt the value of daily rituals when I started to travel more. Teaching a sunset class up a mountain in Oman, as the goats returned home, their bells tinkling, is perhaps my favourite location! The more I travelled, the more I recognised that I needed simple rituals throughout the day to 'ground' me. Whether it is my hot water and lime on waking, my mid-morning espresso or the few exercises I always do as the bath is running.

These routines have always helped my body tune into its natural circadian rhythms. These mini workouts designed for each part of the day – morning, midday, evening – will help you tune into your body, becoming part of your commitment to being more active throughout the day.

We cannot always wake with the dawn, but perhaps you can set your alarm at the same time each morning, allowing yourself an extra 10 minutes for your morning workout. Before breakfast is ideal, otherwise you will need to leave time to digest your breakfast before you work out. For the same reason, it would be best to do your midday workout before lunch. Though you could also do midday workouts mid-morning or mid-afternoon. Or all three! There is a whole section on Sit to Stand, Stand to Sit exercises on page 192, which we hope you will find useful at work. There are two types of evening workouts: one focuses on toning, one on relaxing before bedtime. Neither require goats!

While the mini workouts have been designed for different times of day, feel free to mix and match. Every mini workout has 8–10 exercises and is balanced in terms of spinal movements: spinal flexion, rotation, side flexion and extension. We have done our best to ensure most joints are mobilised to keep you flexible, and key muscles targeted to keep you strong. We have also included one specific breathing exercise in every workout except the Strength and Flexibility Workouts, where we needed the time to warm you up! You always have the option of adding Deep Abdominal Breathing (page 57) at the start and finish. It is up to you to decide how many repetitions to do for each exercise. Everyone works at their own pace.

We timed ourselves and we managed to finish all the workouts within 10 minutes, but we appreciate we are Pilates professionals and know the exercises well. Recognise that it may take you a while to become familiar enough with them to hit the 10 minutes mark, but perseverance (the only prize I ever seemed to win at school) pays off.

You will find our sample Mindful Pilates exercise on page 198. At the end of the Morning Workouts, you will find a section with Tips for Exercising Outdoors (page 185).

Note: You may notice that not every exercise in the book is in the workouts below. Some exercises were simply to teach you the movement skills you need to do the more complex exercises.

Finally, always listen to your body, it is your best teacher and guide. There will be times when you need rest rather than exercise. A walk rather than a workout.

Morning Workouts

Designed to wake you up and energise you for the day ahead. Choose mat-based workouts or standing workouts.

Mat Workouts

WORKOUT ONE

01/ Relaxation Position: Chin Tucks and Neck Rolls (page 40)
02/ Cross Over Shoulder Drops (page 72)
03/ Hip Rolls with Arm Circles (page 111)
04/ Curl Ups with Double Knee Openings (page 141)
05/ Split Stance Cat (page 81)
06/ Dart into Side Bend into Rest Position (page 120)
07/ Rest Position Back Breathing (page 98)
08/ High-kneeling Advanced Side Reach (page 162)
09/ Ski Squats (page 152)

WORKOUT TWO

01/ Relaxation Position Nose Spirals (page 125)
02/ Spine Twirls (page 126)
03/ Curl Ups with Knee Fold and Extension (page 140)
04/ Side Stretch Lying (page 102)
05/ Diamond Press (page 90)
06/ Rocking Cat into Rest Position (page 142)
07/ Side-lying Bow and Arrow (page 86)
08/ Standing Chest Expansion (page 104)
09/ Roll Downs (page 93)

WORKOUT THREE

01/ Relaxation Position: Rainbow Necks (page 124)
02/ Knee Rolls, Knee Openings and Zig Zags (page 67)
03/ The Wave (page 138)
04/ Hip Rolls with Rib Rolls (page 110)
05/ Oyster (page 70)
06/ Cobra Prep into Rest Position (page 91)
07/ Table Top Leg Stretch (page 145)
08/ Standing Side Reach (page 89)
09/ Standing Angel Wings Breathing (page 100)

WORKOUT FOUR

01/ Seated 360/Hundred Breathing (page 99)
02/ Relaxation Position: Chin Tucks and Neck Rolls (page 40)
03/ Spine Curls with Ribcage Closure (page 78)
04/ Spine Curls with Windows (pages 78 and 127)
05/ Oblique Curl Ups (page 108)
06/ Hundred Stage 3 (if possible) (page 176)
07/ Dart into Side Bend into Rest Position (page 120)
08/ Threading the Needle Stretch (page 113)
09/ Ski Squats (holding balance) (page 152)

WORKOUT FIVE

01/ Relaxation Position: Rainbow Necks (page 124)
02/ Staggered Spine Curls with Arm Circles (page 78)
03/ Curl Ups with Double Knee Openings (page 141)
04/ Cobra Prep with Arm Slide and Single Heel Kick (page 168)
05/ Rocking Cat into Rest Position (page 142)
06/ Seated Bow and Arrow (page 87)
07/ High-kneeling Advanced Side Reach (page 162)
08/ Standing Chest Expansion (page 104)

WORKOUT SIX

01/ Standing Breathing Rib Shifts (page 101)
02/ Relaxation Position: Knee Rolls, Knee Openings and Zig Zags (page 67)
03/ Spine Curls with Ribcage Closure (page 79)
04/ Hip Rolls with Rib Rolls (page 110)
05/ Dart into Side Bend (page 120)
06/ Split Stance Cat into Rest Position (page 81)
07/ Standing Windows into Openings Doors (page 128)
08/ Walking on the Spot Squats (page 151)

WORKOUT SEVEN

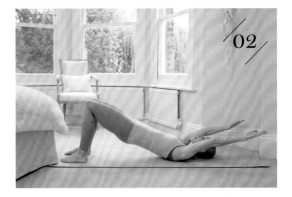

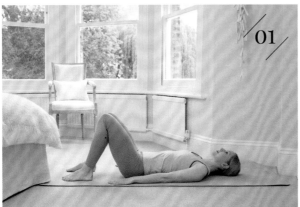

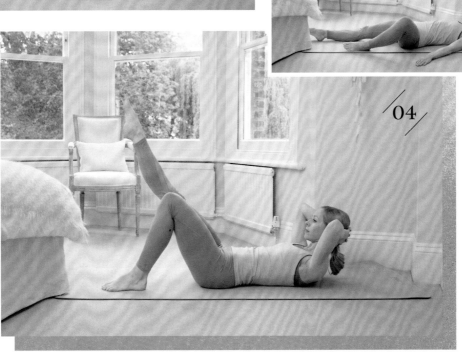

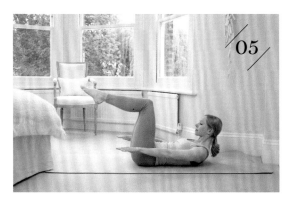

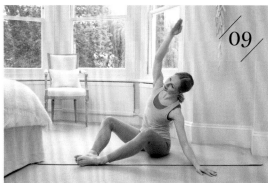

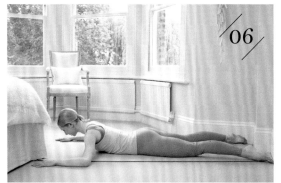

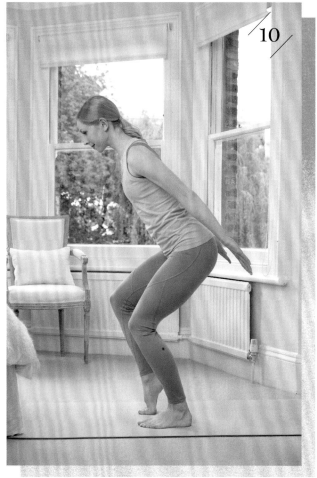

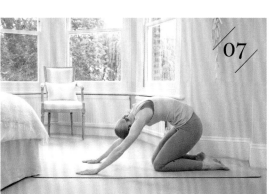

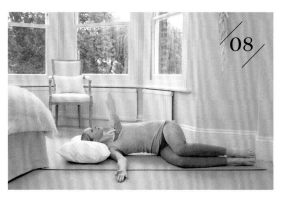

Standing Workouts

You will find more Standing Workouts in the Midday section (page 186). You will notice that Standing Cat appears in most of these workouts. No apologies, it is simply a wonderful way to get your spine and hips moving.

WORKOUT ONE

01/ Standing Angel Wings Breathing (page 100)
02/ Walking on the Spot x2 (page 132)
03/ Standing Cat x2 (page 83)
04/ Split Stance Bow and Arrow x3 (page 87)
05/ Static Lunge with Chest Expansion x2
      (page 157)
06/ Standing Side Reach x 2 (page 89)
07/ Standing Windows x3 (page 128)
08/ Roll Downs x2 (page 93)

WORKOUT TWO

01/ Standing Breathing Rib Shifts (page 101)
02/ Walking on the Spot Squats (page 151)
03/ Split Stance Waist Twists (page 106)
04/ Standing Cat (page 83)
05/ Opening Doors with Flexion and Extension
      (page 116)
06/ Standing Side Reach (page 89)
07/ Dynamic Lunges with Ribcage Closure
      (page 160)
08/ Standing: Box Breathing (page 96)

WORKOUT THREE

01/ Standing One Lung Breathing (page 97)
02/ Walking on the Spot (page 132)
03/ Ski Squats (page 152)
04/ Standing Cat (page 83)
05/ Split Stance Arm Circles with Twist (page 107)
06/ Standing Side Reach (page 89)
07/ Opening Doors with Flexion and Extension
      (page 116)
08/ Dynamic Lunges with Chest Expansion
      (pages 104 and 160)

WORKOUT ONE

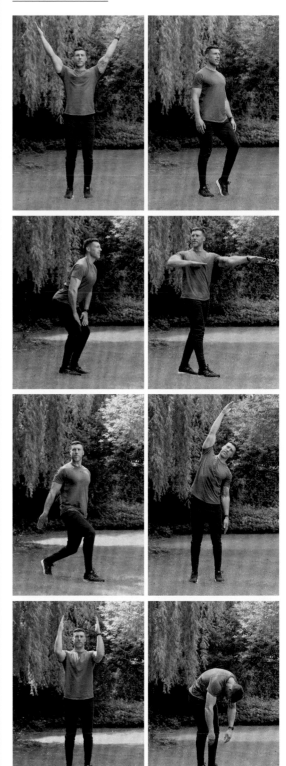

Tips for Exercising Outdoors

Joseph Pilates was passionate about taking recreational activities outdoors, preferably wearing as little as possible to allow the fresh air and sunlight to reach you.

• Wherever possible, take your mat outside or choose an aerobic activity to do outside. A brisk walk through the woods is preferable to a brisk walk on a treadmill (and it's free!). Cycling outdoors is better than a stationary bike, lawn tennis beats squash.

• Whatever the weather, dress appropriately. Wear layers that allow you to move freely and then you can discard them or add more as necessary.

• You may need to wear shoes. If you do, choose shoes with a flexible sole so that you can roll through your feet correctly.

• Try to find flat ground to lay your mat (you may need two), otherwise finding neutral pelvis and spine might be challenging!

• Pick a shady spot. In the warmer months, do not exercise in full sunshine or the heat of the day, even with sunscreen on. When the sun is high, remember to apply a high factor sunscreen before you go out and at regular intervals. If you exercise early morning or later in the afternoon, you can minimise the risk of sunburn or sunstroke. However, in the cooler months, some gentle sunshine is welcome and good for us! If possible, try to get 10 minutes of sunshine every day. This is good for your overall health and especially good for your bones.

• When exercising outdoors, drink plenty of water.

• If you cannot find a suitably flat piece of ground, do the Standing Workouts (page 187).

Midday Workouts

Seated Workouts

One for every working day, assuming that you work a five-day week. Please refer to page 42 for advice about sitting well.

If you are working at a desk, it is a good idea to stand up at least every 30 minutes and walk about to get your circulation going. To help, we have made standing up and sitting down exercises! See page 192. In the meantime, you will find three types of workouts below: Seated, for when you really are tied to your chair; Standing and Sit to Stand, Stand to Sit.

WORKOUT ONE

01/ Seated Angel Wings Breathing (page 100)
02/ Seated Speedy Warm-up (page 137)
03/ Seated Cat (page 82)
04/ Seated Windows into Opening Doors (page 127 and 115)
05/ Seated Waist Twist (page 85)
06/ Seated Chest Expansion (page 104)
07/ Seated Side Reach (page 89)
08/ Seated Vagal Tone Breathing (page 97)

WORKOUT TWO

You will notice One Arm Opening Doors in this workout. Remember, you will need to control your spinal rotation (that is, you should try to prevent it!).

01/ Seated One Lung Breathing x2 (page 97)
02/ Seated Speedy Warm Up x2 (page 137)
03/ Seated Side Reach x2 (page 89)
04/ Seated Knee Rolls x2 (page 68)
05/ Seated One Arm Opening Doors x2 (page 115)
06/ Seated Bow and Arrow x3 (page 87)
07/ Seated Cat x2 (page 82)
08/ Box Breathing x1 (page 96)

WORKOUT THREE

01/ 360 degrees Hundred Breathing (page 99)
02/ Seated Single Floating Arms (page 74)
03/ Seated Walking on the Spot (page 133)
04/ Seated Knee Openings (page 68)
05/ Seated Cat (page 82)
06/ Seated Waist Twist (page 85)
07/ Seated Side Reach (page 89)
08/ Seated Vagal Tone Breathing (page 97)

WORKOUT FOUR

01/ Seated Breathing Rib Shifts (page 101)
02/ Seated Speedy Warm-up (page 137)
03/ Seated Bow and Arrow (page 87)
04/ Seated Knee Rolls, Knee Openings and Zig Zags (page 68)
05/ Seated Cat (page 82)
06/ Seated Side Reach (page 89)
07/ Seated Windows into Opening Doors (page 128)
08/ Seated Chest Expansion (page 104)

WORKOUT FIVE

01/ Seated Nose Spirals (page 125)
02/ Seated Angel Wings (page 100)
03/ Breathing Seated speedy Warm-Up (page 137)
04/ Seated Waist Twist (page 85)
05/ Seated Cat (page 82)
06/ Seated One Arm Opening Doors (page 115)
07/ Seated Side Reach (page 89)
08/ Box Breathing (page 96)

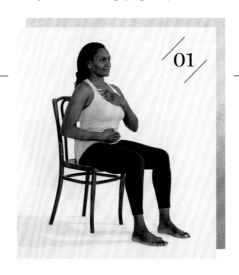

/01/

Standing Workouts

WORKOUT FOUR

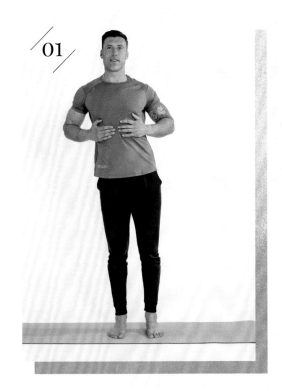

01/

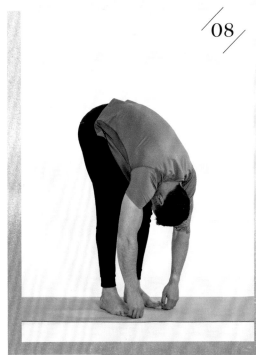

08/

WORKOUT FIVE

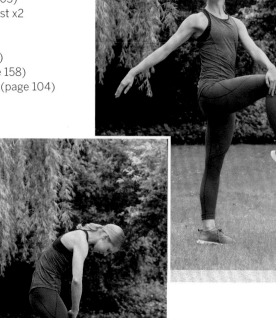

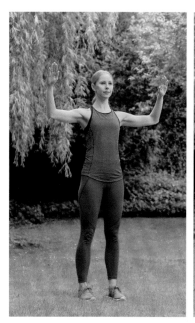

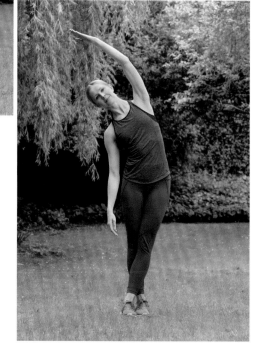

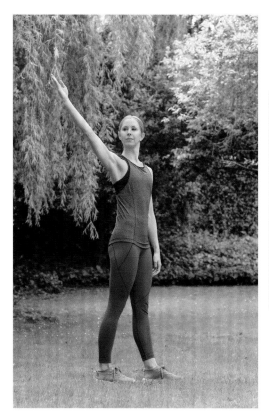

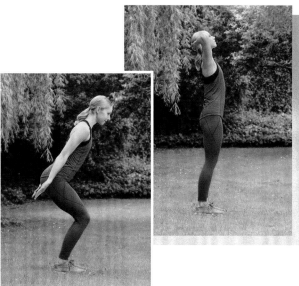

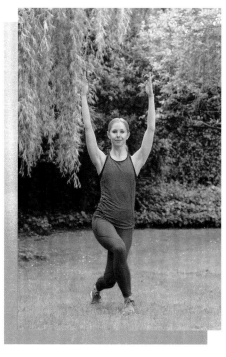

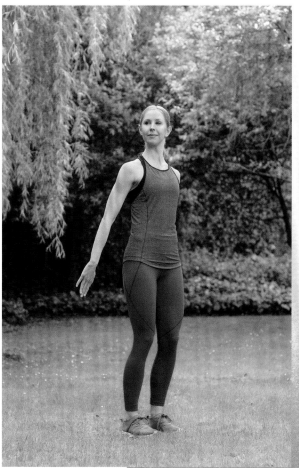

Sit to Stand/ Stand to Sit (STS)

Five workouts here, which include both sitting and standing exercises and, most importantly, the means to get from one to the other. The gluteal muscles are essential in the Sit to Stand manoeuvre. These large muscles are one of the key skeletal muscles that release myokines (hormones) during exercise. During muscle contraction, myokine secretes into the blood system and helps to fight inflammation as well as metabolic diseases, such as diabetes and obesity.[22]

Before we start, we need to establish exactly how you are going to get up and get back down again. Be kind to yourself when trying these workouts. Practice makes perfect but, if you are still finding it difficult, you can place a cushion under your bottom (although remove it for the Seated Exercises) to raise you up or use a higher chair. Note: Workout Five is the hardest. Your chair must be steady and not able to slide away.

Sit to Stand

Start by 'walking' your bottom forwards to the front of the chair. Take a moment and check your postural alignment.

QUICK REMINDER:

- Head balanced centrally on top of the spine.
- Ribcage over pelvis.
- Spine with its natural curves.
- Shoulders open and relaxed.
- Weight even on both sitting bones.

STARTING POSITION

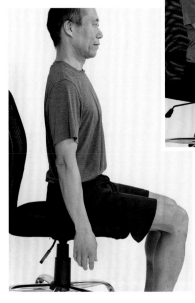

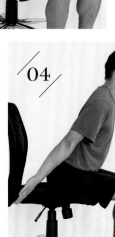

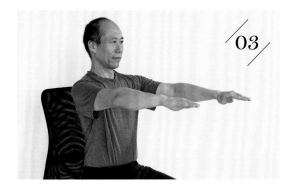

ARM POSITIONS

Your arm position can vary, you can:

01/ Have your arms lengthened by your sides.

02/ Cross your arms over your chest, ensuring collarbones are still wide. (I find this hardest.)

03/ Extend your arms out in front of you, just below shoulder height.

04/ Start with the arms by your sides, palms facing inwards or backwards, then as you stand up, you press back. We can call this Ski Squat arms.

The one thing we do not want you to do is use the arm rests to push up – that's cheating.

FOOT POSITIONS

There are several foot positions possible, depending on what we are challenging in the exercise.

01/ Keep your feet in line with your knees, in line with your hips. Remember the good lower leg alignment we showed you on page 32.

02/ Feet hip-width apart, parallel and fully grounded.

03/ Feet hip-width apart, parallel, one with heel raised.

04/ Feet moved slightly back under the chair, which will bring you onto the balls of both feet.

05/ One foot slightly behind the other in a split stance, on the ball of the back foot.

06/ For when we want to challenge you more, we will ask you to transfer your weight onto one foot. It is too difficult to STS on one leg, so instead we will ask you to lift one heel to bring the weight onto the ball of your foot (and toes). Then transfer some of your weight onto the other foot; the one that is planted fully on the ground. When you stand (or sit back down), this 'planted' foot will be the one you press up/down from.

07/ Spread your toes wide and use them.

08/ We will be asking you to alternate which foot you take back as you STS, to ensure you work both legs evenly.

09/ Once you are Standing, we may change your foot position and, because we know it is complex, we will give you clear directions in italics.

Apologies, we know we are being pedantic about your foot position, but it makes all the difference.

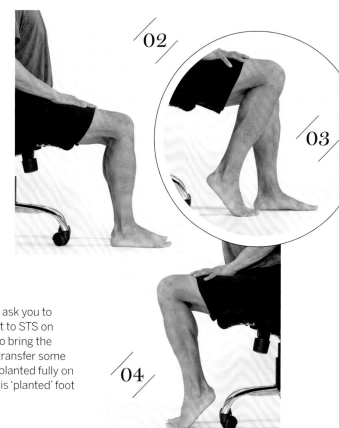

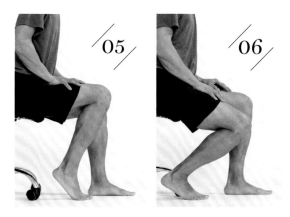

Finally, the **Hip Hinge** and **Sit to Stand**. A full description of Hip Hinge is on page 71. A quick reminder below.

- You are moving your lengthened spine in one 'straight' (but still with its natural curves) piece.

- Stay in control of the line of your head, ribcage and pelvis.

- Do not drop your head or tip it back.

- You are hinging forwards from the hips.

- From the Hip Hinge, it is **Nose over Toes** before you press up into a Squat position. It will not be possible to stand up unless you get your nose over toes.

- We want you to use your gluteal muscles as much as possible to power you up, rather than your thigh muscles (although these will work too!). So, bring your awareness to them and remind them to do the work! If that does not work, you can squeeze them on the way up.

Stand to Sit

The same advice for Sit to Stand applies to Stand to Sit, but this time your thigh muscles work eccentrically; lengthening out as you descend. Sitting down can be harder because it is tougher on your knees. This makes it even more important that your leg alignment is correct so that your patella (kneecap) 'tracks' correctly. When working properly, the kneecap glides in a groove that is near the end of your thigh bone. If the tracking is off, even slightly, it can cause pain and swelling. You will need a lot of control to lower yourself down slowly and precisely. When you are doing the STS/STS workouts, you can repeat the STS/STS manoeuvre or just do it once. When trying the Split Stance versions, swap feet to do repetitions with the other foot forwards and vary which foot you place forwards first, to avoid 'favouring' one foot over the other. Because you will be varying your foot position, when you Stand to Sit again, do make sure the chair is still there before you sit back down!

WORKOUT ONE

Start with feet hip-width and parallel.
01/ Seated Cat (page 82)
02/ Seated Speedy Warm-up (page 137)
Move your right foot back and raise the heel.
03/ Hip Hinge to Stand (page 71). Repeat the STS/STS manoeuvres up to x 6, alternating which foot is back. Then stay up... Split Stance.
04/ Split Stance Arm Circles with Twist (swap feet after 4 reps) (page 107)
Feet parallel and shoulder-width apart.
05/ Standing Side Reach (page 89)
Feet hip-width again.
06/ Walking on the Spot (page 132)
Take the left foot back and heel raise.
07/ Ski Squat to sit back down again, with control. Repeat STS/STS in Ski Squat position x 4.
08/ Seated Box Breathing (page 96)
Next time you do this workout, change the left/rights.

WORKOUT TWO

Start with feet hip-width and parallel.
01/ Seated Windows into Opening Doors (page 128)
Raise your left heel. Transfer your weight onto your right foot.
02/ Hip Hinge to Stand (page 71). Repeat STS/STS manoeuvres up to x6, alternating which foot is back. Then stay up...
Both feet grounded now, hip-width apart.
03/ Standing Cat (page 83)
04/ Walking on the Spot Squats (page 151)
05/ Standing Bow and Arrow (page 87)
Cross feet over for ...
06/ Standing Side Stretch
Hip-width again, raise your right heel, transfer your weight onto your left foot.
07/ Squat to Sit down. Repeat STS/STS Squat x 4.
08/ Seated Vagal Tone Breathing (page 97)
Next time you do this workout, change the left/rights.

WORKOUT THREE

You are getting the hang of this now.
01/ Seated Chest Expansion (page 104)
02/ Seated Speedy Warm-up (page 137)
Take your right foot back and raise the heel. Keep your weight even between both feet this time.
03/ Cross your arms, Hip Hinge to Stand (page 71).
Feet parallel, hip-width apart
04/ Standing Cat (page 83)
05/ Dynamic Lunges with Arm Circles (page 160)
Feet shoulder-width apart.
06/ Standing Side Reach (page 89)
Feet hip-width again.
07/ Standing Waist Twist (page 85)
Take your left foot back and raise the heel. Weight even between both feet.
08/ Cross your arms, Squat to sit back down.
Next time you do this workout, change the left/rights.

WORKOUT FOUR

01/ Seated Box Breathing (page 96)
02/ Seated Speedy Warm-up (page 137)
Feet parallel, right heel raised, transfer most of your weight onto your left foot.
03/ Hip Hinge to Stand (page 71). Repeat STS/STS manoeuvres up to x 6 alternating which foot is back.

Both feet grounded.
04/ Standing Bow and Arrow (page 87)
Cross feet over for
05/ Standing Side Stretch
Feet hip-width and parallel again.
06/ Squats with Chest Expansion (page 104 and 150)
07/ Standing Cat (page 83)
Feet parallel, left heel raised, transfer most of your weight onto your right foot.
08/ Squat to Sit. Repeat the STS/STS manoeuvres up to x 6 alternating which foot is back.
Next time you do this workout, change the left/rights.

WORKOUT FIVE

A slightly longer and more challenging workout.
01/ Seated 360/Hundred Breathing (page 99)
02/ Seated Walking on the Spot (page 133)
Take your right foot back and raise the heel. Keep the weight even between both feet.
03/ Hip Hinge to Stand (page 71) but this time pause halfway. Hold the position (but not your breath)... 1 ...2....3....4....5...... Stand up.
Repeat STS/ STS manoeuvres up to x 3 alternating which foot is back.
Split Stance.
04/ Split Stance Waist Twists (swap feet after 4 reps) (page 85)
Feet parallel, hip-width apart.
05/ Standing Cat (page 83)
Feet shoulder-width.
06/ Standing Side Reach (page 89)
Feet hip-width.
07/ Standing Angel Wings Breathing (page 100)
Take your left foot back, raise the heel.
08/ Squat to Sit... wait for it...pause half-way... 1...2...3...4...5... Sit down. Repeat the STS/STS manoeuvres up to x 6 alternating which foot is back.
09/ Seated Vagal Tone Breathing (page 97)
Next time you do this workout, change the left/rights

> *Moving on...* Once you are confident you can Sit to Stand and Stand to Sit in perfect alignment, you could also add an arm action.
>
> **FOR EXAMPLE:** Ribcage Closure (page 73), Arm Circles (page 76), Angel Wings Breathing (page 100) Or... Add a balance: as you are coming up, raise up onto your toes.

WORKOUT THREE

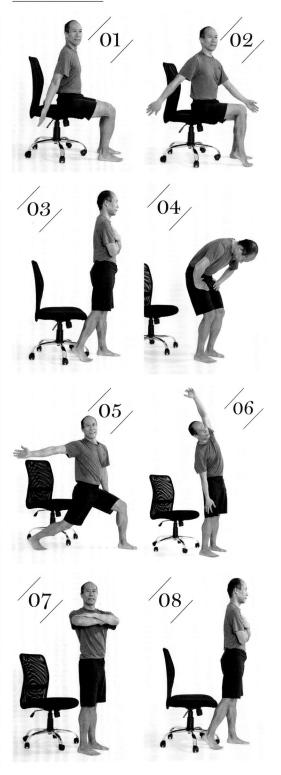

Evening Workouts

There may be evenings when you want to work harder, focusing on your strength and flexibility. Or if you have had a tough day, you might simply want a relaxing, calming workout. We have catered for both.

Strength and Flexibility Workouts

WORKOUT ONE

01/ Relaxation Position: Chin Tucks and Neck Rolls (page 40)
02/ Spine Curls with Arm Circles (page 78)
03/ Hip Rolls (page 88)
04/ Oblique Curl Ups (page 108)
05/ Prep for Roll Up (page 172)
06/ Single Leg Stretch (page 171)
07/ Cobra into Rest Position with Back Breathing (pages 170 and 98)
08/ Side-kick Series (page 148)
09/ Mermaid with Rib Rolls (page 118)
10/ Dynamic Lunges with Ribcage Closure (pages 160 and 73)

WORKOUT TWO

01/ Relaxation Position: Rainbow Necks (page 124)
02/ Spine Curls with Windows (pages 78 and 127)
03/ Spine Twirls (page 126)
04/ Roll Up or Prep for the Hundred (page 174 and 172)
05/ Chair Lifts (page 149)
06/ Cobra Prep with Arm Slide and Heel Kicks into Rest Position (page 168)
07/ Table Top Taps (page 144)
08/ High-kneeling Advanced Side Reach (page 162)
09/ Split Stance 'Curtsy' Squats (page 158)
10/ Roll Downs (page 93)

WORKOUT THREE

01/ Squats with Ribcage Closure (page 73)
02/ Relaxation Position: Nose Spirals (page 125)
03/ The Wave (page 138)
04/ Hundred (page 176)
05/ Side-lying Bow and Arrow (page 86)
06/ Dart with Salute into Side Bend (page 121)
07/ Split Stance Cat into Rest Position (page 81)
08/ Rest Position with Back Breathing (page 98)
09/ Back Bridge with Dips (page 165)
10/ Dynamic Lunges with Chest Expansion (pages 160 and 104)

WORKOUT FOUR

01/ Relaxation Position: Nose Spirals (page 125)
02/ Spine Curls with Ribcage Closure (pages 73 and 78)
03/ Oblique Curls with Rib Rolls (page 109)
04/ Single Leg Stretch (page 171)
05/ Side Press-ups (page 175)
06/ Oyster (page 70)
07/ Dart into Star (page 166)
08/ Rocking Cat into Rest Position (page 142)
09/ Mermaid (page 117)
10/ Walking on the Spot Squats (page 151)

WORKOUT FIVE

01/ Relaxation Position: Chin Tucks and Neck Rolls (page 40)
02/ Spine Curls with Arm Circles (pages 78)
03/ Hip Rolls with Rib Rolls (page 110)
04/ Roll Up or Prep for the Hundred (pages 174 or 172)
05/ The Hundred (page 176)
06/ Dart with Salute into Side Bends (page 121)
07/ Rocking Cat into Rest Position (page 142)
08/ Single Leg Pull Front Prep (page 147)
09/ Split Stance Arm Circles with Twist (page 107)
10/ Roll Downs (page 93)

WORKOUT SIX

01/ Relaxation Position: Chin Tucks and Neck Rolls (page 40)
02/ Spine Curls with Arm Circles (pages 78 and 76)
03/ Curl Ups with Double Knee Openings (page 141)
04/ Roll Up or Prep for the Hundred (page 174 and 172)
05/ Cobra into Rest Position (page 170)
06/ Advanced Threading the Needle (page 114)
07/ Back Bridge with Dips (page 165)
08/ Chair Lifts (page 149)
09/ Standing Side Reach (page 89)
10/ Dynamic Lunges with Ribcage Closure (pages 160 and 73)

WORKOUT SEVEN

01/ Standing Chest Expansion (page 104) x2
02/ Walking on the Spot Squats (page 151) x2
03/ The Wave (page 138) x2
04/ Hundred (page 176) x2
05/ Dart with Salute into Side Bend (page 121) x2
06/ Rocking Cat into Rest Position (page 142) x4
07/ Single Leg Pull Front Prep (page 147) x3
08/ Static Standing Lunge with Waist Twists
　　(pages 53 and 85) x2
09/ Roll Downs (page 93) x2

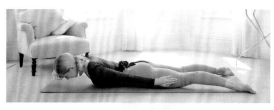

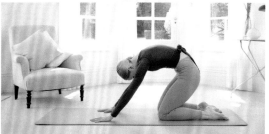

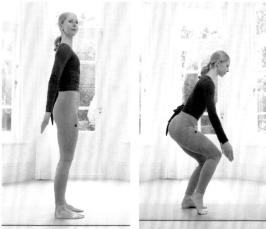

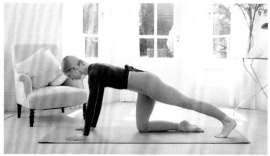

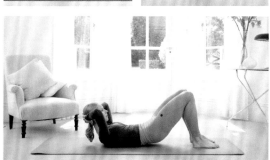

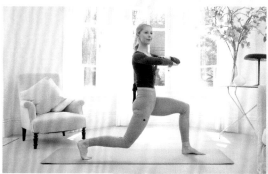

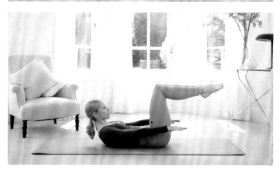

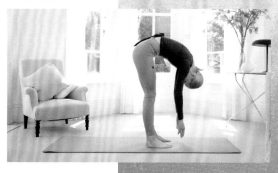

Relaxing Workouts

Perfect before bedtime. At the end of this section, you will find tips on how to ensure a good night's rest.

WORKOUT ONE

01/ One Lung Breathing (page 97)
02/ Shoulder Drops (page 72) x2
03/ Spine Curls with Arm Circles (pages 78 and 76) x2
04/ Hip Rolls with Rib Rolls (page 110) x2
05/ Cat into Rest Position (page 80 and 98) x2
06/ Threading the Needle Stretch (page 113) x2
07/ High-kneeling Advanced Side Reach (page 162) x 2
08/ Roll Downs (page 93) x2

WORKOUT TWO

01/ Standing Angel Wings Breathing (page 100)
02/ Long Frog Mermaid (page 117)
03/ Relaxation Position: Nose Spirals (page 125)
04/ Spine Twirls (page 126)
05/ Cobra Prep (page 168)
06/ Split Stance Cat into Rest Position (pages 81 and 98)
07/ Rolling Chalk Circles (page 130)
08/ Relaxation Position: Vagal Tone Breathing (page 97)

WORKOUT THREE

01/ Relaxation Position: Rainbow Necks (page 124)
02/ Spine Curls with Ribcage Closure (page 79 and and 73)
03/ Knee Rolls, Knee Openings and Zig Zags (page 67)
04/ Hip Rolls with Rib Rolls (page 110)
05/ Dart with Salute (page 121)
06/ Cat into Rest Position (pages 80 and 98)
07/ Side Kick Series: Front and Back (page 148)
08/ Side Stretch Lying... add Vagal Tone Breathing (page 102 and 97)

WORKOUT FOUR

01/ Relaxation Position: Neck Rolls and Chin Tucks (page 40)
02/ Knee Rolls, Knee Openings and Zig Zags (page 67)
03/ Spine Curls with Split Stance (page 79)
04/ Diamond Press (page 90)
05/ Cat into Rest Position with Back Breathing (page 80)
06/ Rolling Chalk Circles (page 130)
07/ Seated Side Reach (page 89)
08/ Seated Vagal Tone Breathing (page 97)

WORKOUT FIVE

01/ Relaxation Position: Windows (page 127)
02/ Spine Curls Twirls (page 126)
03/ Knee Rolls, Knee Openings and Zig Zags (page 67)
04/ Full Star (page 146)
05/ Rocking Cat into Rest Position (page 142)
06/ Side-lying Bow and Arrow (page 86)
07/ Mermaid (page 117)
08/ Seated or Relaxation Position: One Lung Breathing (page 97)

WORKOUT SIX

01/ Ribcage Closure with Leg Slide (pages 73 and 63)
02/ Knee Folds and Extension (page 65)
03/ The Wave (page 138)
04/ Cobra Prep with Arm Slide and Heel Kicks into Rest Position (page 168)
05/ Threading the Needle Stretch (page 113)
06/ Seated Side Reach (page 89)
07/ Rolling Chalk Circles (page 130)
08/ Relaxation Position: Angel Wings Breathing (page 100)

WORKOUT SEVEN

01/ Relaxation Position: Cross Over Shoulder Drops (page 72)
02/ Spine Curls with Arm Circles (page 78)
03/ Hip Rolls with Rib Rolls (page 110)
04/ Side-Kick Series Front and Back (page 148)
05/ Diamond Press (page 90)
06/ Cat into Rest Position (pages 80 and 98)
07/ Mermaid (page 117)
08/ Seated or Relaxation Position: Vagal Tone Breathing (page 97)

WORKOUT ONE

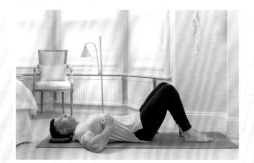

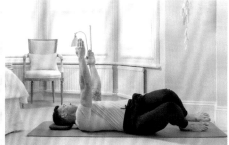

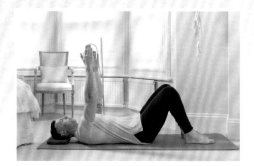

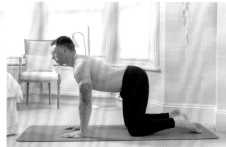

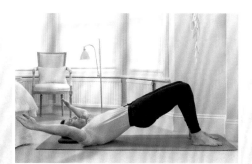

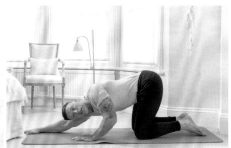

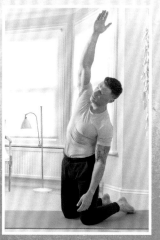

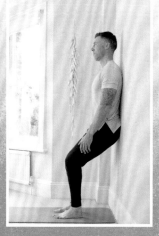

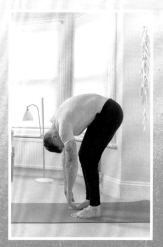

Mindful Pilates Practice

Below, you will find an example of one exercise, Spine Curls, which has Mindfulness added to the directions. You could take the same 'formula' and apply to other exercises, such as Hip Rolls (page 88), Side Reach (page 89), Waist Twists (page 85), Cat (page 80) or Standing (page 50). We would recommend a simple version of an exercise, rather than the more complicated combination exercises, so that you do not have to worry about what to do next.

We suggest you record the directions or you can try one of the Mindfulness sessions on our online subscription channel:
www.bodycontrolpilatescentral.vhx.tv

Here, I wish to give my wholehearted thanks to my dear friend and colleague, Brenton Surgenor (Senior Lecturer Dance Science, The Hong Kong Academy for Performing Arts), who helped develop our Mindful Pilates technique.

SPINE CURLS WITH MINDFULNESS

Use all your senses; listen, watch, smell, taste, feel, sense, lock yourself into the present moment. Relaxation Position (page 37). Feet grounded, kneecaps floating towards the ceiling. Arms lengthened by your sides, palms down.

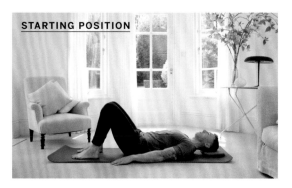

STARTING POSITION

Bring your awareness to your mind.

NOTICE:

• the quality of your mind.
• any thoughts or feelings you might be having.

Without judgement, notice your thoughts and feelings in this moment.

Bring your awareness to your breath.

NOTICE:

• the rhythm of your breath.
• the moments between the inhalation and exhalation.
• which parts of your body move on the in-breath and which move on the out-breath.

Without judgement, notice your breathing in this moment.

Bring your awareness to your body.

NOTICE:

• the weight of your body on the floor.
• which parts of your body are heavy into the floor and which parts are light and away from the floor.

Without judgement, notice your body in this moment.

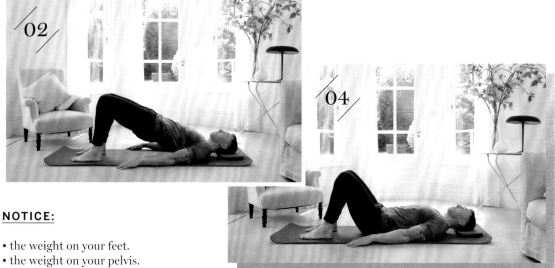

NOTICE:

- the weight on your feet.
- the weight on your pelvis.
- the weight on your ribcage.
- the weight on your head.

Do you notice any tension? Do you feel balanced? Think about any changes you might like to make to your alignment. Observe where you are now and, with self-kindness, gently direct your body to release residual tension and to feel more balanced.

Bring your awareness to your movement.

01/ Take a slow, easy in-breath and bring your awareness to your pelvis.

02/ As you breathe out, curl the tailbone off the floor and roll the spine up, bone by bone, to the bottom of your shoulder blades, until your knees are in line with hips and shoulders.

03/ Take an easy in-breath and bring your awareness to the length of the body from shoulders to hips and knees. Notice the weight of your feet on the floor and the relationship of the knees to the hips and the feet.

04/ As you breathe out, slowly curl back down, lengthening out the spine, bone by bone, until you have returned to the Starting Position.

What sensations have you observed in your body as you moved? After each repetition, are you aware of the same sensations or do these sensations change? Make a mental note of these sensations and any changes.

Repeat steps 1–4 until you have completed two full Spine Curls.

Bring your awareness back to your body.

NOTICE:

- Your body on the floor and any sensations in your body.

Without judgement, notice the sensations in your body and make a mental note of these sensations. Bring your awareness back to your breath.

NOTICE:

- the quality of your breath and whether your breathing has changed from the beginning of the exercise.

Without judgement, notice your breathing in this moment.

Bring your awareness back to your mind.

NOTICE:

- the quality of your mind and any thoughts and feelings.

Without judgement, notice your thoughts and feelings in this moment.

Working Your *Heart*

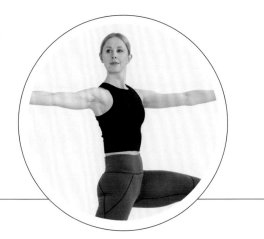

Like any muscle, your heart needs to be worked regularly to keep it healthy and this means doing cardiovascular exercise. Although Pilates is a fabulous body conditioning method, it is not a cardiovascular workout. The only notable exception would be the Hundred and some of the Dynamic Lunges and Squats where the arms are used too. To ensure good heart health, you need to add some cardiovascular activities to your weekly routine.

A cardiovascular or aerobic activity is one which moves your whole body, especially if it involves the large muscles like the legs. During cardiovascular or aerobic exercise, oxygen is needed to power your muscles. As you become aerobically fit, your body becomes more efficient at transporting oxygen.

Cardiovascular activities have many other major health benefits, they:

- strengthen the heart, lungs and circulatory system.
- reduce the risk of heart disease.
- reduce blood pressure.
- improve blood cholesterol and triglyceride levels.
- release endorphins, the feel-good hormones, which in turn reduces stress levels and may help with depression.
- improve muscle strength.
- improve weight management.

WORLD HEALTH ORGANIZATION 2020 GUIDELINES ON PHYSICAL ACTIVITY & SEDENTARY BEHAVIOUR

For **adults aged 18–64**, without medical issues, the WHO recommends 150–300 minutes of moderate intensity aerobic physical activity or 75–150 minutes of vigorous intensity a week. We should also do muscle-strengthening activities that involve all major muscle groups on two or more days. This is longer than previous recommendations. If you are

over 65, there is no let up, the amount is the same, and they add functional balance and strength training on at least three days per week to prevent falls and improve your body's overall function.

For **children and adolescents**, the guidelines are per day rather than per week. Recommending an hour of moderate to vigorous intensity daily, along with muscle-strengthening activities at least three times a week. And **babies** need to get 30 minutes of tummy time daily!

This is a lot of physical activity. But don't despair, you can add a considerable amount of aerobic activity incrementally during your day, in the same way as you have added muscle strengthening with the workouts. (See pages 202–3 for tips.)

MODERATE AEROBIC ACTIVITY

- brisk walking
- water aerobics
- riding a bike on level ground or with few hills
- doubles tennis
- pushing a lawn mower
- hiking
- skateboarding
- rollerblading
- volleyball
- basketball
- dancing

VIGOROUS AEROBIC ACTIVITY

- jogging or running
- swimming fast
- riding a bike fast or on hills
- singles tennis
- squash
- football
- rugby
- skipping
- hockey
- aerobics
- gymnastics
- martial arts

INCIDENTAL AEROBIC ACTIVITIES

You need to decide what works best for you. It can be a mix of moderate and vigorous, incidental, or planned. However, in line with our Pilates Express® approach to keep you moving throughout the day, we recommend you incorporate as many incidental aerobic activities (see pages 202–3) as possible. To keep yourself motivated, be sure to choose activities that you enjoy.

WORKING AT THE RIGHT INTENSITY

It is important when doing cardiovascular exercise that you keep track of your heart rate. You will need to work out your resting heart rate first. This is the number of times your heart beats per minute when you are at rest. A good time to check it is in the morning after you've had a good night's sleep and before you have a cup of tea or coffee!

For most of us, 60–100 beats per minute (bpm) is normal. However, the rate can be affected by factors like stress, anxiety, hormones, medication, and how physically active you are. If you're fit, your heart rate will be lower, as your heart muscle is in better condition and doesn't have to work as hard to maintain a steady beat.

TO WORK OUT YOUR HEART RATE:

• Take your pulse on the inside of your wrist, on the thumb side.

• Use the tips of your first two fingers (not your thumb) and press lightly over the artery.

• Count your pulse for 30 seconds and multiply by two to find your beats per minute.

The table below shows target heart rate zones for different ages. Your maximum heart rate is about 220 minus your age. Look at the age category closest to yours and read across to find your target heart rates. Target heart rate during moderate intensity activities is about 50–70 per cent of maximum heart rate, while during vigorous physical activity it is about 70–85 per cent of maximum. The figures are averages, so use them as a general guide.

If you have a Fitness Tracker, it will do the calculations for you! If your heart rate is too high, you're working too hard. If it's too low, and the intensity feels 'light' to 'moderate', you may want to push yourself to exercise a little harder, especially if you're trying to lose weight. If you've been inactive for a while, aim for the lower range of your target zone (50 per cent) and gradually build up. In time, you will be able to exercise comfortably at up to 85 per cent of your maximum heart rate.

AGE	TARGET HEART RATE ZONE (50–85%)	AVERAGE MAX HR (100%)
20 years	100–170 bpm	200 bpm
30 years	95–162 bpm	190 bpm
35 years	93–157 bpm	185 bpm
40 years	90–153 bpm	180 bpm
45 years	88–149 bpm	175 bpm
50 years	85–145 bpm	170 bpm
55 years	83–140 bpm	165 bpm
60 years	80–136 bpm	160 bpm
66 years	78–132 bpm	155 bpm
60 years	75–128 bpm	150 bpm

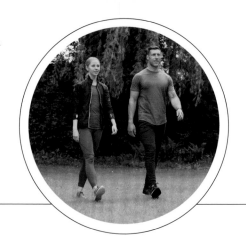

Incidental Exercise ——
Step by Step

There are endless ways you can add incidental exercise to your day. One way is to increase the number of steps you take per day; 4,000 steps a day (spread throughout the day) will start the improvement in your health. You will need to do 7,000 steps to improve your fitness and a total of 10,000 steps per day to lose weight.

You will need to ensure that you are walking at a fast enough pace to raise your heart rate for your walking to count as an aerobic activity. This means a gentle stroll in the park is not enough, your pace needs to be brisk enough to raise your heart rate. You should bear in mind that, even if you meet your 10,000 steps a day, you may still fall short of the required amount of cardio activity to maintain heart health. The good news is that counting your steps is incredibly easy. Most mobile phones have an app you can download which will log your steps and you can also count your steps and check your cardio activities on a Fitness tracker watch. There are some very good ones on the market that do not cost the earth.

LET'S WALK BETTER

It has been calculated (by SnowBrains.com) that, during the average lifetime, we take over 216 million steps, walking about five times around the equator! Walking is free, low impact and has been proven to be good, not just for our physical, but our mental health too.

Just like Breathing, Standing, Sitting, and Sit to Stand, Stand to Sit, there are ways we can improve our walking by being mindful and conscious of how we are walking. Please bear in mind that we all have our own individual gait, but there are a few simple things you can do to help improve how you walk.

- Firstly, ensure that you are wearing supportive footwear, preferably with a flexible sole that allows you to roll through the foot. A good pair of shoes will make all the difference; they need to cushion your feet and support your ankles to prevent injury.

- Try not to carry bags as they restrict your arm movements and can add uneven load to the body. If you must carry a bag, backpacks carried centrally work best. Otherwise, at least alternate which shoulder you carry the bag on to balance you out.

- Posture. Always, always, walk tall. No slouching. But beware of 'fixing' your posture... shoulders relaxed rather than pulled back. While we do not want your abdomen to protrude, it is not feasible to engage your core muscles for any length of time as you walk and trying to do so may restrict your movements. One of the goals of this programme is to encourage your deep core muscles to work naturally, without conscious effort and to have lasting endurance to help you maintain good posture throughout the day. In the meantime, perhaps take a moment before you set off to stand tall, head over ribcage, ribcage over pelvis, shoulders relaxed and down. Gently connect to your core muscles to remind yourself... then relax them as you walk. You can always remind yourself every so often.

- Allow your arms to swing in a low arc naturally rather than trying to 'pump' them, which can create unnecessary tension. Your arm arc will become larger as you walk faster.

- With each step, allow the arm opposite your forwards foot to swing straight forwards, not diagonally across the body. Then as your forwards foot comes back, the opposite arm swings back straight. Allow your ribcage and pelvis to rotate naturally and easily as you walk.

- Look ahead, rather than down (unless you are traversing over very difficult terrain). Looking down puts enormous strain on your neck and upper spine. Focus your eye about 10–20 feet ahead of you; your head will follow the direction of your eyes.

- Foot action. Try to strike the ground first with your heel, then roll through the foot from heel to toe, before pushing off again from the base of your toes on your back foot to propel you forwards. Note: it is very important to maintain flexibility at the base of your big toes to enable you to push off correctly. If this joint becomes locked, it can upset your gait and potentially your back too. We have been working on this throughout the programme, whenever we asked you to rise onto your toes for example, with Ski Squats with Heel Raises on page 152, we have been encouraging flexibility and stability of the feet and ankles. The hip, knee and ankle alignment we have been working on throughout the programme will also help you to roll through the feet properly… neither rolling in or out.

- Try not to make your stride too wide, as this can stress your lower leg joints.

- Pace. The first few minutes of your walk should be at a gentle, even, comfortable pace and then you can gradually speed up. Ideally, at this stage you should still be able to carry on a conversation without becoming breathless. If you are able, you can then increase your pace to be moderately intense, which should affect your breathing so that you start to breathe harder (but not so hard that you cannot talk). Try to maintain this moderately intense pace for about 30 minutes. Then, you can start to ease off the pace, gradually slowing it down. Spend about 10 minutes at the slower pace to allow your heart rate to settle.

- If time and circumstances permit, do a few Pilates Express® exercises before and after your walk. One of the Standing Workouts would be ideal, or if you've only time for a couple, try: Standing Speedy Warm-up (page 134); Standing Cat (page 83) Split Stance Arm Circles with Twists (page 107); Ski Squats with Heel Raises (page 152).

And now, some suggestions on how to increase your number of steps:

- Try parking furthest away from, rather nearest, the station, shops or office.

- Walk rather than take the underground or bus or at least get off a stop earlier and walk the rest of the way.

- Similarly, walk to the furthest bus stop or tube station.

- Take the stairs rather than the lift.

- If there is an escalator, walk rather than stand on it. You can also walk on the moving walkways at airports.

- During your lunch break, try walking around the block a few times before you eat your lunch.

- Take short breaks at work by running your own errands.

- If you have a mobile phone, walk around as you talk.

- Rather than sending an email, go and talk to your colleague.

- Buddy up with a friend to help make it fun.

- Play active, rather than sedentary, video games.

- Play active games with your children and/or grandchildren. Tag is timeless!

Finally, let us allow the UK's Chief Medical Officers to have the final word:

'The good news is that even small changes can make a big difference over time…some is good, more is better…. You always feel better for being active. We want as many people as possible to protect their future health and start their journey to a healthier life now.'

Further Information

For more information on Body Control Pilates, for local teachers, classes, teacher training courses, books and equipment, please visit www.bodycontrolpilates.com

If you have enjoyed the exercises and workouts in this book, you will love Body Control Pilates Central, our online video subscription channel. You will find Pilates Express® workouts presented by Lynne and Sarah, as well as masterclasses, workouts, tutorials and lots more for the public and teachers alike. Please visit www.bodycontrolpilatescentral.vhx.tv

Follow us on Facebook:
www.facebook.com/BodyControlPilates
Follow us on Instagram:
@bodycontrolpilates and **@bcpcentral**
Follow us on Twitter: **@bodycontrol**

Our Body Control Pilates flagship studio and headquarters is based in Bloomsbury, central London. You can visit us and the Rosetta Stone at The British Museum all in one trip!

The Body Control Pilates Centre
35, Little Russell Street
London WC1A 2HH
Tel:+44 (0)20 7636 8900
Email: info@bodycontrol.co.uk

CARDIOVASCULAR ACTIVITIES

For information on heart health, visit The British Heart Foundation's website: **www.bhf.org.uk**

This US website also has lots of sound advice on cardiovascular activities: **www.heartorg.com**

THE GREAT OUTDOORS: SUNLIGHT, DAYLIGHT, FRESH AIR

For information on your local Forest Schools, please visit: **www.forestschoolassociation.org**

NUTRITION

Helen Ford is Head of Nutrition at Glenville Nutrition Clinic.

www.glenvillenutrition.com
Email: reception@glenvillenutrition.com
Tel: + 44 (0)1892 515905
Instagram: @helenfordnutrition

OBESITY & EATING DISORDERS

For the British Nutrition Foundation visit:
www.nutrition.org.uk

If you are worried about obesity, visit the British Obesity Society: **www.britishobesitysociety.org**.

The National Health Service website **www.nhs.uk** has some great advice about obesity.

So too does the US website **www.obesity.org.**

For information on eating disorders you can visit:
www.beateatingdisorders.org.uk
www.nationaleatingdisorders.org
www.nhs.uk/conditions/Eating-disorders

STRESS

If your stress is becoming overwhelming, do consult your doctor, and you may like to visit Stress Management Society: www.stress.org.uk

If you are interested in meditation, visit British Meditation Society: **www.britishmeditationsociety.com**

SLEEP

If you are having trouble sleeping and feel it is affecting your health, speak to your doctor. The NHS website has advice on insomnia: **www.nhs.uk/conditions/insomnia**

References

1. UK Chief Medical Officers' Physical Activity Guidelines, September 2019
2. 'Breaking sitting with light activities vs structured exercise: a randomised crossover study demonstrating benefits for glycaemic control and insulin sensitivity in type 2 diabetes.' Bernard Duvivier,et al, Diabetologia, March 2017
3. World Health Organization 2020 Guidelines on Physical Activity and Sedentary Behaviour
4. 'Daily sit to stands performed by adults: a systematic review', R. W. Bohannon, Journal of Physical Therapy Science 27 , March 2015
5. 'Joint association of physical activity and body mass index with cardiovascular risk: a nationwide population-based cross sectional study', P.L. Valenzueala et al., The European Journal of Preventative Cardiology, January 2021
6. 'Vagal-immune interactions involved in cholinergic anti-inflammatory pathway', Zila I. et al, Physiological Research, Czech Academy of Sciences, 2017
7. 'Humming greatly increases the amount of nasal nitric oxide', Eddie Weitzberg et al, American Journal of Respiratory and Critical Care Medicine, 2002
8. 'Irritable Bowel Syndrome: The effect of FODMAPS and meditation on pain management', Shannon M. Cearley, European Journal of Integrative Medicine, June 2017
9. 'Meditation for post traumatic stress: Systemic review and meta-analysis', Lara Hilton et al, Psychological Trauma, 2017
10. 'Evidence based Non Pharmacological Therapies for Fibromyalgia', Mansoor M Aman et al., Current Pain and Headache Reports, 2018
11. 'Effects of transcendental meditation on trait anxiety: a meta-analysis of randomised controlled trials', David W. Orme-Johnson et al, The Journal of Alternative and Complementary Medicine, 2014
12. 'Observing the Effects of Mindfulness-Based Meditation on Anxiety and Depression in Chronic Pain Patients', Kim Rod., Psychiatria Danubina, 2015
    'Meditation programs for psychological stress and well being; a systematic review and meta- analysis', Madhav Goyal et al, JAMA Internal Medicine, 2014
    'Mindfulness, meditation may ease anxiety, mental health stress', Harvard Health Publishing January 8, 201
    'Daily Stress and the benefits of mindfulness: Examining the daily and longitudinal relations between present-moment awareness and stress responses', James N Donald, Journal of Research in Personality, 2016
    'How Positive Emotions build Physical Health: Perceived Positive Social Connections account for the upward spiral between Positive Emotions and Vagal Tone', Bethany E, KOK, Kimberley A Coffey Michael, Cohn et al, Sage Journals Psychological Science, 2013
13. 'If we can regulate our breathing, we can initiate a state of calm, or get ready for action we can increase capacity for alertness', Gerbarg and Brown, 2016
    'Yoga therapy for Anxiety', Pilkington, Karen, Gerbarg, P.L, Brown R. P, Principles and practice of yoga in health care, Handspring Publishing
    'The role of deep breathing on stress', Valentina Perciavalle et al, Neurological Sciences, March 2017
14. 'Contraction of the human diaphragm during postural adjustments', Hodges P. et al, Journal of Physiology, 1997
    'Changes in intrabdominal pressure during postural and respiratory activation of the human diaphragm', Hodges P., Journal of Applied Physiology, 2000
15. Paul W. Hodges 'Postural activity of the diaphragm is reduced in humans when respiratory demand increases', The Journal of Physiology, December 2001
    Hold it sister – The confident girl's guide to a leak free life, Mary O'Dwyer
16. Proceeds of the National Academy of Sciences, August 2016.
17. 'Overtraining effects on immunity and performance in athletes', Laurel T MacKinnon, Immunology & Cell Biology, Volume 78 Issue 5, 2000
    'The immune system and overtraining in athletes: clinical implications', Anthony C Hackney et al, Acta Clinica Croatica, 2012
18. Center for Disease Control and Prevention
19. 'Impact of insufficient sleep on total daily energy expenditure, food intake and weight gain', Rachel R. Markwald et al, Proceedings of the National Academy of Sciences of the USA, 2013
20. 'The relationship between insomnia, sleep apnoea and depression: findings from the American national health and Nutrition Examination Survey 2005-2008', A. C. Hayley et al, Australian & New Zealand Jouranl of Psychiatry, 2015
21. 'Revised estimates for the Number of Human and Bacteria Cells in the Body Ron Sender', Shai Fuchs and Ron Milo, Published online, PLOS Biology, August 2016
    'A human gut microbial gene catalogue established by metagenomic sequencing', Junjie Qin et al, Nature, 2010
    'The Integrative Human Microbiome Project: dynamic analysis of microbiome-host omics profiles during periods of health and disease', Integrative HMP (iHMP) Research Network Consortium Cell Host Microbe, 2014
    'Gut microbiota, obesity, and diabetes', Elaine Patterson et al, Postgraduate Medical Journal, May 2016
22. 'Induced Myokines in Muscle Homeostasis and the Defence against Chronic Diseases', Claus Brandt and Bente K. Pedersen, BioMed Research International, March 2010

Index

Acknowledgements

You'd think that after writing 18 books I'd have run out of things to say! As a constant learner, I find that there are always new things to share - this book itself was conceived before, but written during, the coronavirus pandemic. The pandemic changed all our priorities and, as a result, the book's content evolved. I found myself researching how Pilates can help you to improve immune and respiratory health and reduce stress. I ended up writing enough for two books!

Thank you, Michael and Judith for your wise steerage; the team at Kyle Books for editing my manuscript into a publishable book; Emma at Studio Nic&lou for designing a book which has room to breathe; Claire for your stunning, sensitive photography.

Zoom helped me to develop the programme with my dear friend and colleague, Sarah. Sarah's creativity is only matched by her eye for alignment. She can spot a misplaced joint blindfolded from 10 paces! I'd be lost without her on both a personal and professional front.

The photo shoot took place in difficult circumstances with strict adherence to Covid-secure guidelines. Bless the models who bravely volunteered to take part. Thank you so much to all of you for your patience and fortitude:

Freya Field (freyafield@hotmail.co.uk)
Tunde Olayera (tundepilates.co.uk)
Chantal Pilbrow (thankupilates.com/)
Jon Ashton (www.ashtonpilates.com)
Remigiusz Kubas (Instagram: kubas_boxing_academy)
Derek Chow (www.restorebalancepilates.com)
Daniel Dewhurst (instagram.com/dan_does_pilates/

I am also indebted to my clients, in particular the lovely Linda who tested all of the new exercises.

Body Control Pilates would not have survived without our incredible tutor and office team. And, as for our Body Control Pilates community - 1,500 teachers, several hundred students, and many tens of thousands of clients - the collective support throughout the pandemic was beyond anything we could have imagined when we set up Body Control Pilates over 25 years ago! I thank you.

And finally, whilst my Pilates work is my passion, I am above all a proud mother and an even prouder Nanny. I am blessed to have such a wonderful loving family. Welcome to our newest grandson Henry, born during the pandemic, and already a charmer. Watch out world! If we could only bottle his laugh as medicine. Amy and Evie, you bring joy, beyond measure, with everything you do.

I wish health and happiness to each, and every one of you, family, friends, colleagues, teachers, clients and readers.

Bio

Lynne Robinson is one of the world's most recognised and respected Pilates teachers. She is the Founder of the Body Control Pilates organisation, whose education programme is seen as an international benchmark for safe, effective teaching. Lynne is perhaps best known through her best-selling books, including *The Pilates Bible*, *Pilates for Life*, *Shape Up the Pilates Way* and DVDs. Her teaching has regularly taken her as far afield as Japan, Hong Kong, Australia, the Middle East and the USA.

An Hachette UK Company
www.hachette.co.uk

First published in Great Britain in 2022 by
Kyle Books, an imprint of
Octopus Publishing Group Limited
Carmelite House
50 Victoria Embankment
London EC4Y 0DZ
www.kylebooks.co.uk
www.octopusbooksusa.com

ISBN: 9780857839237

Text copyright © Lynne Robinson 2022
Design and layout copyright © Octopus Publishing
Group Limited 2022
Photography copyright © Claire Pepper 2022

Distributed in the US by Hachette Book Group, 1290 Avenue of the Americas, 4th and 5th Floors, New York, NY 10104

Distributed in Canada by Canadian Manda Group, 664 Annette St., Toronto, Ontario, Canada M6S 2C8

Lynne Robinson has asserted her right under the Copyright, Designs and Patents Act 1988 to be identified as the author of this work.

All rights reserved. No part of this work may be reproduced or utilised in any form or by any means, electronic or mechanical, including photocopying, recording or by any information storage and retrieval system, without the prior written permission of the publisher.

Publishing Director: Judith Hannam
Publisher: Joanna Copestick
Design: Emma Wells, Studio Nic & Lou
Photography: Claire Pepper
Editor: Jenny Dye
Editorial Assistant: Zakk Raja
Production: Lisa Pinnell

A Cataloguing in Publication record for this title is available from the British Library

Printed and bound in China

10 9 8 7 6 5 4 3 2 1